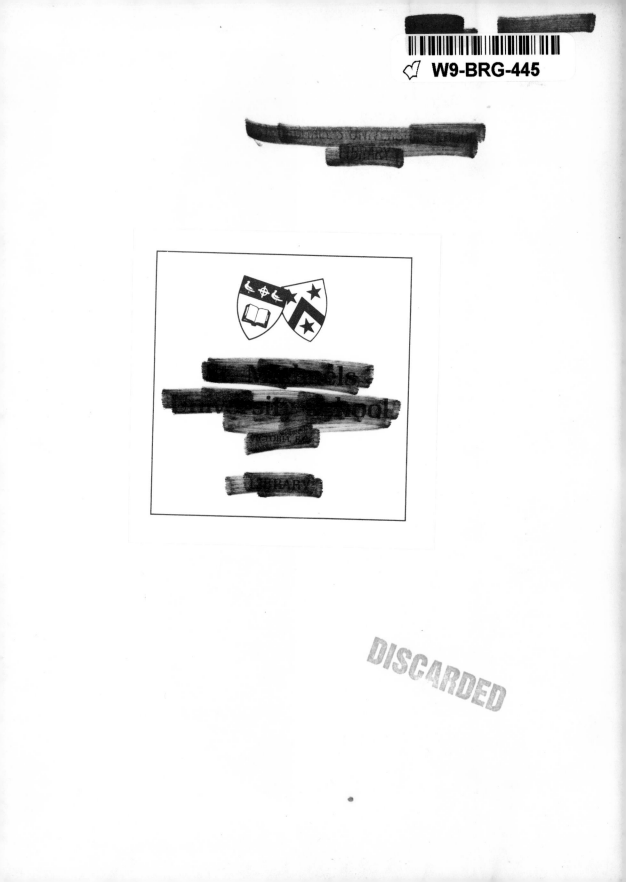

PREGNANCY

—— AND ——

CHILDBIRTH

THE ILLUSTRATED BOOK OF

PREGNANCY

— AND —

CHILDBIRTH

Margaret Martin

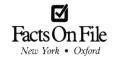

Facts On File

New York • Oxford

The Illustrated Book of Pregnancy and Childbirth
Text and Illustrations copyright © 1991 by Margaret Martin

Facts On File, Inc.   Facts On File Limited
460 Park Avenue South   Collins Street
New York NY 10016   Oxford OX4 1XJ
USA   United Kingdom

Library of Congress Cataloging-in-Publication Data
Martin, Margaret, 1954-
    The illustrated book of pregnancy and childbirth / Margaret
Martin.
        p. cm.
    Includes index.
    ISBN 0-8160-2570-3
    1. Childbirth. 2. Pregnancy. I. Title.
RG525.M33   1991
618.2—dc20   91-9050

A British CIP catalogue record for this book is available from the British Library.

Facts On File books are available at special discounts when purchased in bulk quantities for businesses, associations, institutions or sales promotions. Please contact our Special Sales Department in New York at 212/683-2244 (dial 800/322-8755 except in NY, AK, or HI) or in Oxford at 865/728399.

Text design by Donna Sinisgalli
Jacket design by Catherine Hyman
Composition by Facts On File, Inc.
Manufactured by R.R. Donnelly & Sons, Inc.
Printed in the United States of America

10 9 8 7 6 5 4 3 2 1

This book is printed on acid-free paper.

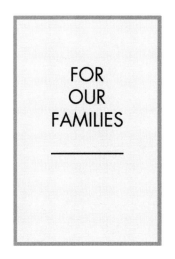

FOR
OUR
FAMILIES

CONTENTS

FOREWORD

I have been teaching childbirth classes for many years. But each new group I meet surprises me by knowing so little about the workings of their bodies, about childbirth, about labor and delivery. There is certainly ample information available in books and magazine articles, and most people have been told in high school or college about the extraordinary engineering feat our bodies perform when we give birth to a child. But in spite of all the information, old wives' tales and misconceptions are passed on from generation to generation, from woman to woman.

Margaret Martin's book fills in the gaps in so many people's knowledge. Her book describes in simple language and with wonderfully clear illustrations what is happening in our bodies when we are expecting a baby. The author tells what to look for in the various stages and phases of labor and delivery, and then continues to discuss the first week postpartum.

She includes a chapter on nutrition, and though many of us know what is meant by "healthy eating," few of us know much about healthy eating once we are pregnant.

Pregnancy and childbirth are considered to be among the peak experiences in a person's life. Both physically and emotionally we need a guide to see us through and help us understand what changes, both physical and emotional are likely to occur.

This book is such a guide for every woman who is expecting a child.

Elisabeth Bing, FACCE

ACKNOWLEDGMENTS

I am deeply grateful to the many hundreds of pregnant women and their families whom I have educated throughout the years, for allowing me to share in their journey through pregnancy and childbirth. This journey, more often than not, brings out the best that men and women have to offer—love, hope, determination, patience, faith, and a generous optimism regarding the future. Sharing in this journey has been an incomparably rewarding adventure.

I must also acknowledge the pioneers of modern birth education, Dr. Grantley Dick Read of England, whose work in the early part of this century was followed by Dr. Fernand Lamaze, in France, and Dr. Robert Bradley, in the United States; Elisabeth Bing, whose vision and tireless efforts are responsible for the training of Lamaze educators throughout the United States through A.S.P.O. (American Society for Psychoprophylaxis in Obstetrics), and Marjie and Jay Hathaway, who, with Dr. Bradley, have worked to train Bradley educators throughout the United States through the A.A.H.C.C. (American Academy of Husband-Coached Childbirth), and who initially trained me.

I warmly thank my husband, my children, and my parents for their patience and loving support.

I affectionately acknowledge Emilie Sparks, Sylvia Solana, Christine Vega, M.P.H., R.D., and Tomi Mikkelsen, whose commitment, friendship, and work helped me bring the Pregnancy and Natural Childbirth Education Center to life in Los Angeles in the late 1970s and early '80s, and Drs. Stephen Brunton, John George, Uziel Reiss, N.B. Ettinghausen, and the other doctors, nurses, and educators who formed the core of the Center's Advisory Board.

I thank Laura Blanchette for her invaluable technical assistance in preparing the copy for this book, and for her patience and unflagging good spirits.

Thanks are due, too, for ongoing inspiration provided by the wonderful staff and students of U.C.L.A.'s School of Public Health, whose dedicated enthusiasm and committed work daily improve both the health and quality of life of individuals and families throughout the U.S. and around the world.

And special thanks go to my friend and mentor, the late Norman Cousins, whose kind interest helped to make the publication of this book a reality.

Education provides options. It makes choices appear where dictates and custom previously ruled. Education adds color and dimension to a black-and-white, two-dimensional view of the world.

Some women have asked me, "Why learn about pregnancy, labor, and birth? It's all just going to happen by itself, anyway!"

And these women are right! Something's going to happen "anyway," that's for sure! The question is what?

The fact that complaints of pregnancy, from headaches and nausea to heartburn, indigestion, constipation, and backache (as well as a host of others), can be prevented entirely, or drastically reduced, is only one reason to learn about pregnancy.

Learning about pregnancy and good prenatal care (including excellent nutrition and exercise) can reduce or eliminate entirely serious risk factors for the child.

Low birth weight (babies born under 5 1/2 pounds), which is associated with about a 300% increase in other birth defects, can often be prevented. Similarly, an educated woman can eliminate many other risk factors, which otherwise could lead to a longer, more difficult labor, birth, and recovery for herself.

Giving birth without knowing what's going on is kind of like going on a roller-coaster ride with a bag over your head. Sure, you get to the end of the ride, all right, but flinging along, without knowing what to expect, can be a frightening, even horrifying experience for the mother.

It's important to realize that the emotions of a woman in labor play a very large part in the progress of that labor. Labor is controlled by hormones released within a woman's body. The release of these hormones is determined to a very large degree by the emotional condition of the laboring woman. If she is frightened and tense, her body can actually work against itself. Labor can slow down. Contractions (of the uterus) can become less effective.

If she is relaxed and in good spirits, her labor can progress more rapidly and easily.

For this reason alone, many doctors today are vigorously recommending that the women they will be attending in childbirth attend classes about pregnancy and birth. They observe an enormous difference in the progress of the labors of educated, relaxed women.

We can be frightened of things we do not understand. Once we understand them, we can manage them, and even enjoy them.

For many women, pregnancy can also be a lonely experience. She is always aware of being pregnant. She cannot move, think, or breathe without that awareness. But it's not so for everyone else. This Illustrated Book makes it easy for every member of the family to understand what's going on in pregnancy, labor, and birth. In this way, the entire family can provide much-needed support and encouragement to the pregnant woman, and better welcome the child.

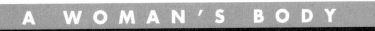

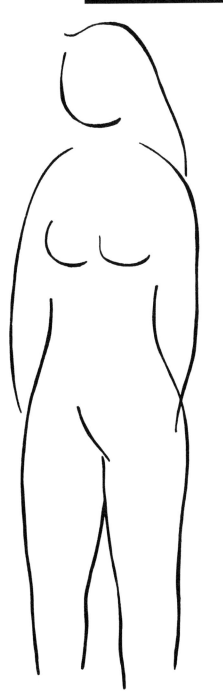

To understand how pregnancy and birth happen, it is necessary to understand a little about a woman's body.

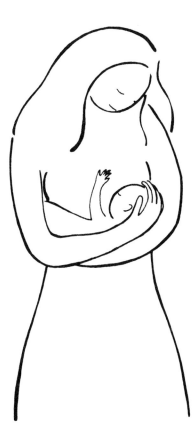

BODY OPENINGS

(1) The URETHRA, the passage leading from the bladder through which urine flows out of the body.

(2) The VAGINA is the passage leading to the uterus.
The VAGINA is also called the BIRTH CANAL. This is because a baby, when ready to be born, must pass from the uterus, through the VAGINA, and out into the world.

(3) The RECTUM is the lowest part of the large intestine. Solid body wastes (bowel movements) pass through this passage and out of the body.

(4) The BLADDER is the little triangle-shaped bag that holds urine, the body's liquid waste.

(5) The UTERUS (WOMB) is the muscle-bag in which a baby grows, shown before pregnancy, when it is about the size of a small pear.

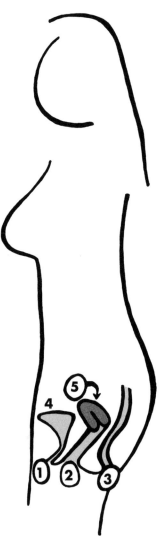

BONES

(6) The PUBIC BONE in the lower front part of the body, which protects the *bladder* behind it.

(7) The SPINE or BACK BONE.

(8) The TAIL BONE is the lowest part of the spine. It is also called the COCCYX.

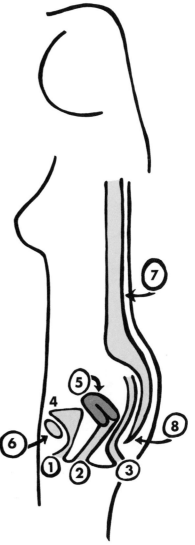

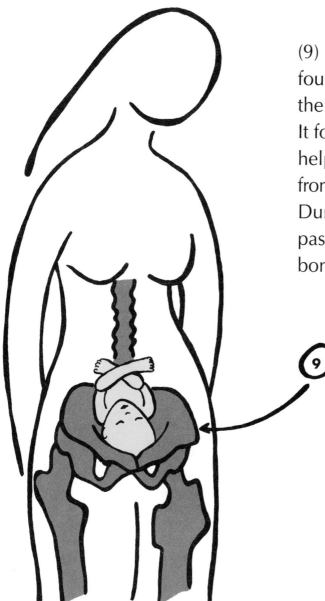

(9) The PELVIS is made of four large bones between the leg bones and the spine. It forms a bony ring that helps to protect the baby from injury during pregnancy. During childbirth, the baby passes through this ring of bones.

MENSTRUATION

The Monthly "Period"

When a girl becomes a young woman, her body prepares itself for the possibility of one day becoming a mother, growing a child within her body, and giving birth to a new being.

Part of this preparation is the growth of her breasts. Other signs are the appearance of hair under her arms and in the pubic area, and the appearance of MENSTRUATION.

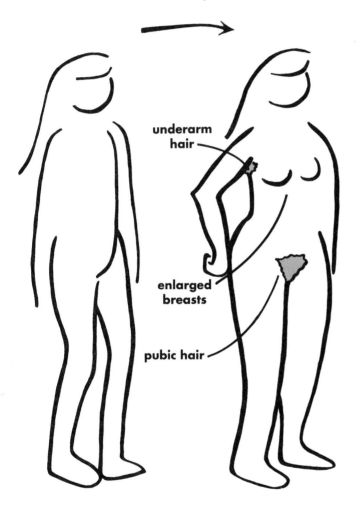

underarm hair

enlarged breasts

pubic hair

GIRL   **YOUNG WOMAN**

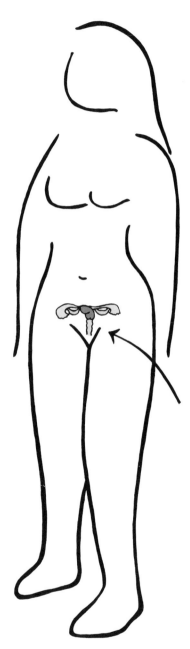

A woman carries eggs (OVA) in two little sacs inside her body called OVARIES. When she is born she already has all the eggs she ever will have.

One OVARY is on either side of the UTERUS (womb). Each OVARY is connected to the UTERUS by a thin TUBE. (FALLOPIAN TUBES—named after Gabriel Fallopius, who first described them.)

OVULATION

Each month one egg ripens and bursts from one of the OVARIES into the FALLOPIAN TUBE. The ovaries take turns. Each one sends out one ripe egg every other month.

OVULATION is the time a ripe egg leaves the OVARY. It occurs only once each month, usually about 10 to 16 days after the first day of the last PERIOD.

The **menstrual period** occurs every 24 to 32 days, and lasts from three to five days. Most women experience 28 day menstrual cycles. (Their menstrual periods occur every 28 days.)

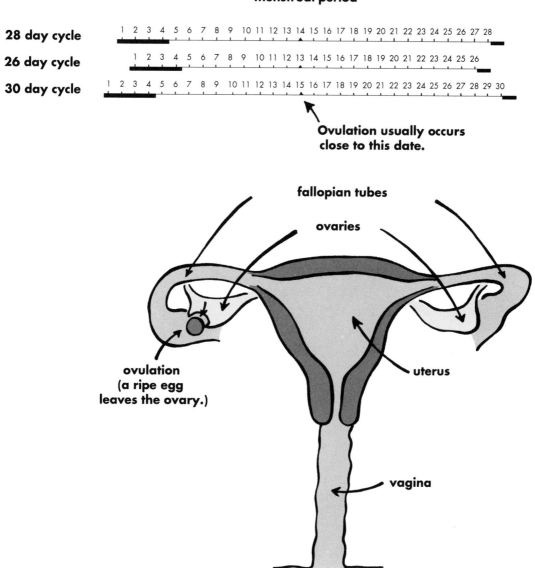

menstrual period

28 day cycle 1 2 3 4 5 6 7 8 9 10 11 12 13 14 15 16 17 18 19 20 21 22 23 24 25 26 27 28

26 day cycle 1 2 3 4 5 6 7 8 9 10 11 12 13 14 15 16 17 18 19 20 21 22 23 24 25 26

30 day cycle 1 2 3 4 5 6 7 8 9 10 11 12 13 14 15 16 17 18 19 20 21 22 23 24 25 26 27 28 29 30

Ovulation usually occurs close to this date.

fallopian tubes

ovaries

ovulation
(a ripe egg
leaves the ovary.)

uterus

vagina

The UTERUS prepares itself for the coming egg by building up layers of menstrual blood inside itself, to nourish the egg.

If the egg is *not* fertilized (does not meet up with a live sperm within about 24 hours after it leaves the OVARY) the egg will deteriorate and the menstrual blood built up inside the UTERUS will fall away—out of the UTERUS, through the VAGINA, and out of the woman's body.

This monthly loss of the unfertilized egg and menstrual blood is called MENSTRUATION, or more commonly, a woman's monthly PERIOD. It occurs about 400 times in a woman's life, beginning in her early teens, and ending sometime 30 to 40 years later.

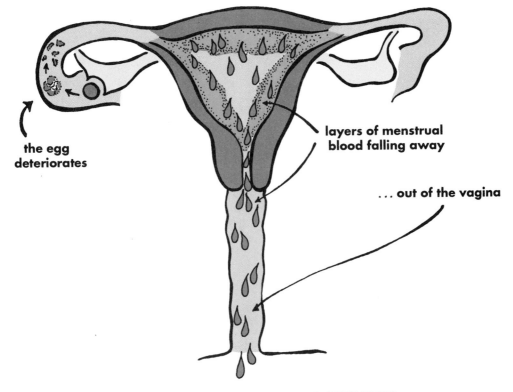

the egg deteriorates

layers of menstrual blood falling away

... out of the vagina

CONCEPTION

When sperm are deposited in or near the opening of the vagina and one of them meets a ripe egg in the Fallopian Tube, CONCEPTION OCCURS.

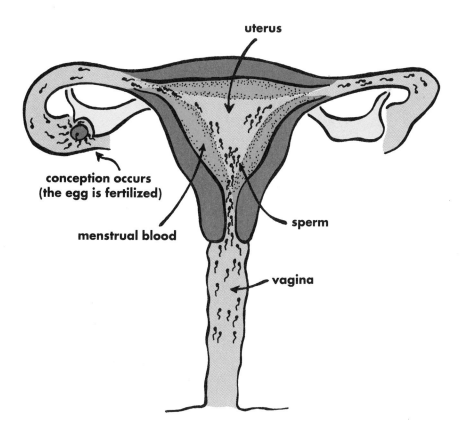

uterus

conception occurs
(the egg is fertilized)

menstrual blood

sperm

vagina

The fertilized egg travels through the Fallopian Tube to the uterus, where it becomes implanted within the menstrual blood, which nourishes it.

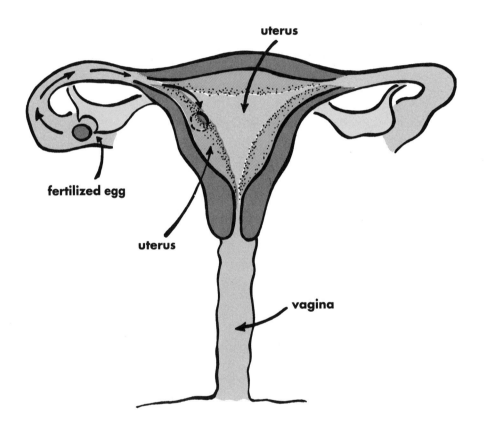

A baby begins to grow inside the woman's uterus. The menstrual blood, instead of being lost, is used to nourish the growing embryo. (An unborn child is called an embryo for the first 2 months.) The woman misses her period, and discovers she is PREGNANT!

TIMING IS IMPORTANT

Timing is important because **conception** will only occur when a sperm meets an egg within about 24 hours after **ovulation**.

However, sperm can remain active for several days inside the uterus waiting for ovulation to occur and an egg to become available for fertilization. This means **a woman can actually become pregnant** (if ovulation occurs) **up to four days after having sexual intercourse.**

Drawings are actual size.

Pregnancy is usually *counted* from the first day of the last menstrual period. However, pregnancy *actually begins* with **conception**, which occurs within a day of **ovulation**, or about 10 to 16 days after the first day of the last period.

Therefore, at 4 1/2 weeks of pregnancy, the baby is usually only about 2 weeks along.

**4 1/2 weeks
(one month)**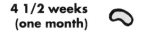

The heart starts beating. The embryo is now about 1/5 inch long. The woman has just missed her menstrual period for the first time, and suspects she may be pregnant.

**9 weeks
(2 months)**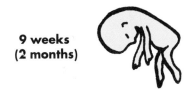

Now the baby is called a fetus, not an embryo. It is basically fully formed. All the parts of a full-term baby are present. The fetus is just over an inch long.

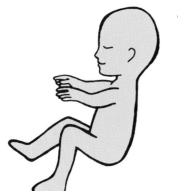

**13 1/2 weeks
(3 months)**

The fetus is about 2 1/2 to 3 inches long. Eyes are closed.

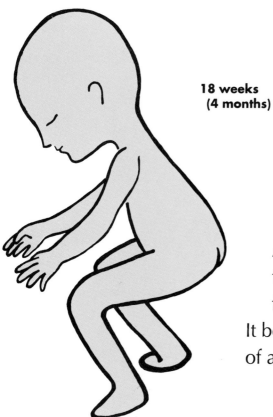

**18 weeks
(4 months)**

Arms and hands are fully formed, with fingernails. The fetus is about 6 inches long. It begins to drink several ounces of amniotic fluid every day.

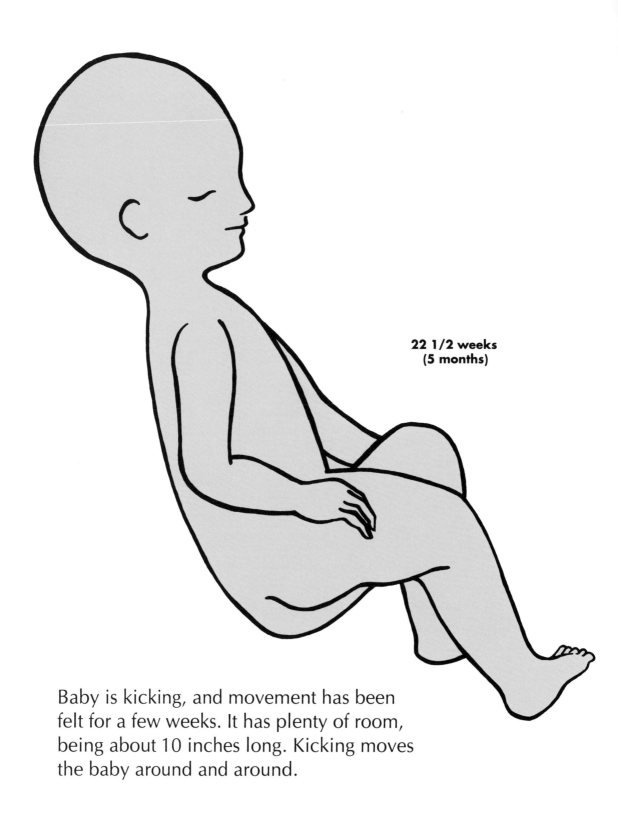

22 1/2 weeks
(5 months)

Baby is kicking, and movement has been
felt for a few weeks. It has plenty of room,
being about 10 inches long. Kicking moves
the baby around and around.

There is less space for the child. It is now over 12 inches long. The baby is very thin. It gains only 1/3 of its birth weight in the first 6 months of pregnancy. Now the baby probably weighs about 2 1/2 pounds.

**27 weeks
(6 months)**

The fetus is usually over 13
inches long

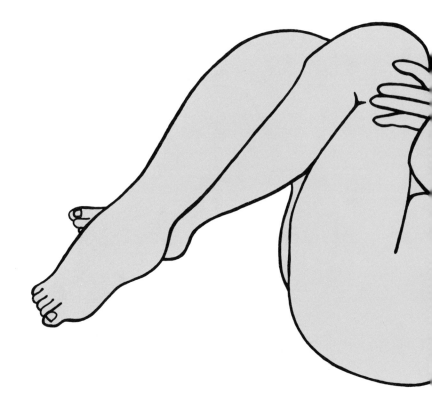

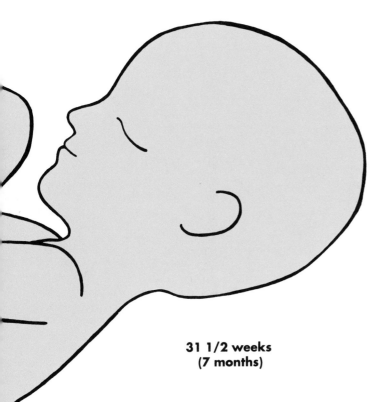

**31 1/2 weeks
(7 months)**

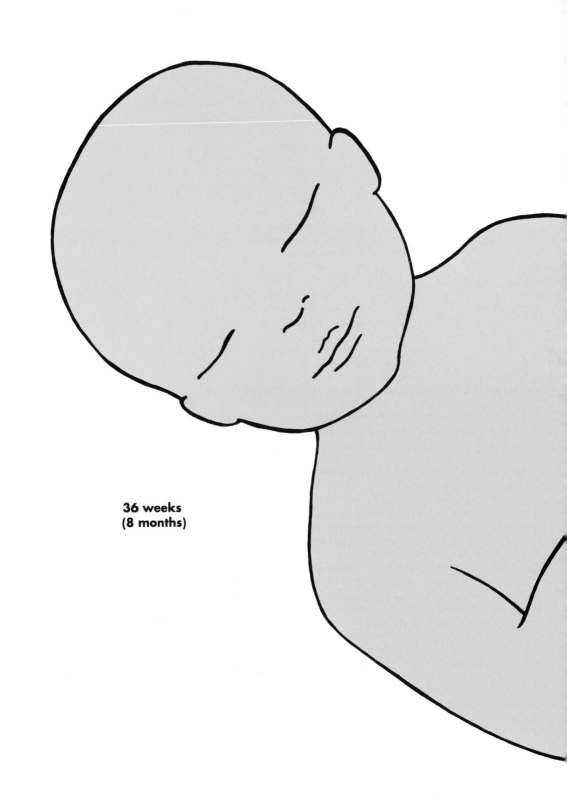

**36 weeks
(8 months)**

The fetus is usually between 15 and 17 inches long. During this month, brain cells form more rapidly than at any other time in a person's whole life. A good diet and enough protein are especially important.

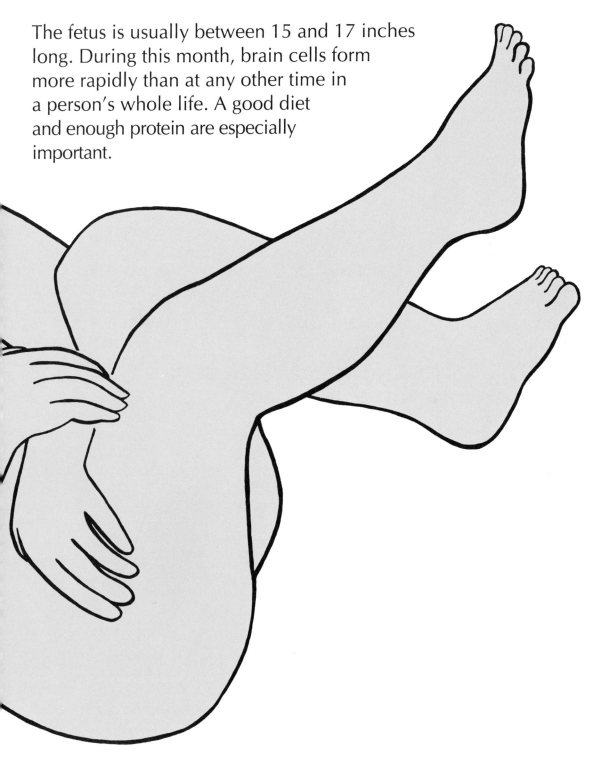

The newborn infant is usually about 20 inches
long (about 1/20 the size of the mother's body).
It can be born at any time between the 266th and
294th day after the first day of the last menstrual period.

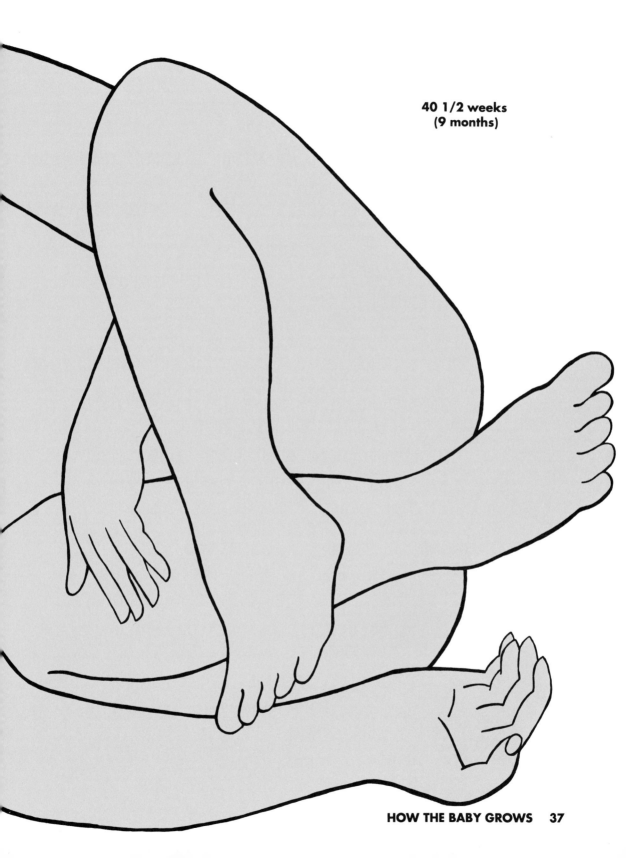

40 1/2 weeks
(9 months)

We have seen *how* the baby grows. In order to understand pregnancy, labor and birth, you must also understand *where* the baby is growing and *what parts* of the mother's body are affected.

The BABY can see, hear, and is recording memories even before it is born.

The AMNION (water bag). The baby is inside a bag-of-waters called the AMNION. It is thin and made of layers. It is filled with amniotic fluid and the baby.
A good diet helps keep the AMNION strong and from breaking too soon.

AMNIOTIC FLUID, often called the "waters." This is the clear, salty fluid that surrounds the baby inside the amnion. From the 4th month on, the baby drinks several ounces of AMNIOTIC FLUID every day. It is part of the baby's food before birth, and helps to cushion and protect the baby during pregnancy.

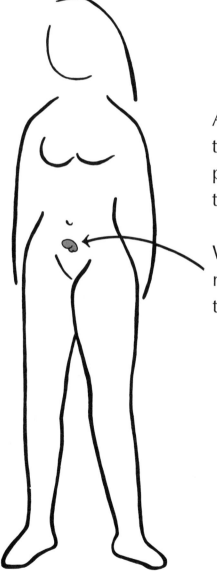

Another bag surrounds
the amnion. It is a very
powerful muscle-bag called
the UTERUS or WOMB.

When a woman is not preg-
nant, the UTERUS is about
the size of a small pear.

During pregnancy, the UTERUS grows to about 20 times its non-pregnant size and becomes very strong. This strong muscle is shaped like a bag and holds and protects the baby.

The opening of the uterus is called the CERVIX. It is much thicker than the sides of the uterus during pregnancy. This is to hold the baby in. The CERVIX is shaped like the neck of a turtle-neck shirt.

(Remember, the UTERUS and its opening, the CERVIX, are all muscle.)

The amnion is connected to the inside of the uterus by the PLACENTA. The word PLACENTA comes from a Latin word meaning flat cake. The PLACENTA is flat and round.

The PLACENTA is the baby's life-support system. Through the PLACENTA the baby receives food and oxygen from the mother's blood. Waste from the baby's body passes into the mother's blood through the PLACENTA. The PLACENTA can be compared to the filter on a fish tank.

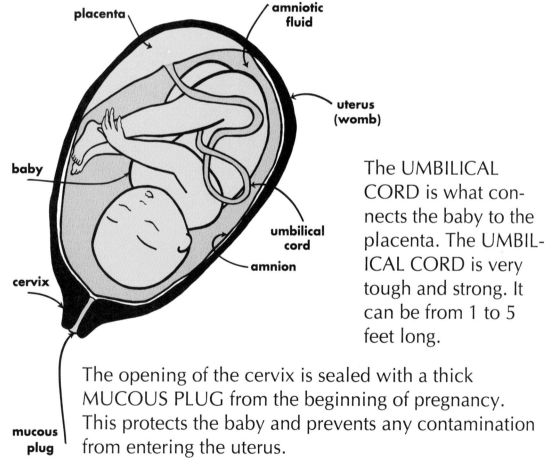

The UMBILICAL CORD is what connects the baby to the placenta. The UMBILICAL CORD is very tough and strong. It can be from 1 to 5 feet long.

The opening of the cervix is sealed with a thick MUCOUS PLUG from the beginning of pregnancy. This protects the baby and prevents any contamination from entering the uterus.

WHAT HAPPENS INSIDE THE WOMAN'S BODY AS THE BABY GROWS?

(1) The ABDOMEN is the middle part of the body. The ABDOMEN contains the stomach, intestines, liver, and other organs.

(2) The STOMACH is the special muscular bag in the abdomen where food that is eaten digests so that the body can make use of it.

(3) The INTESTINES are the long, long tubes that carry food from the stomach through the body, and carry solid wastes (bowel movements) out of the body.

(4) Above the stomach is the LIVER. The LIVER is important in helping the body get good use from food you eat. The LIVER also helps the body get rid of poisons, drugs, or food impurities.

(5) Above the abdomen is the DIAPHRAGM, a muscular wall that separates the abdomen from the chest area.

(6) The HEART is the muscle that pumps blood throughout the body.

(7) The UTERUS lies at the bottom part of the abdomen.

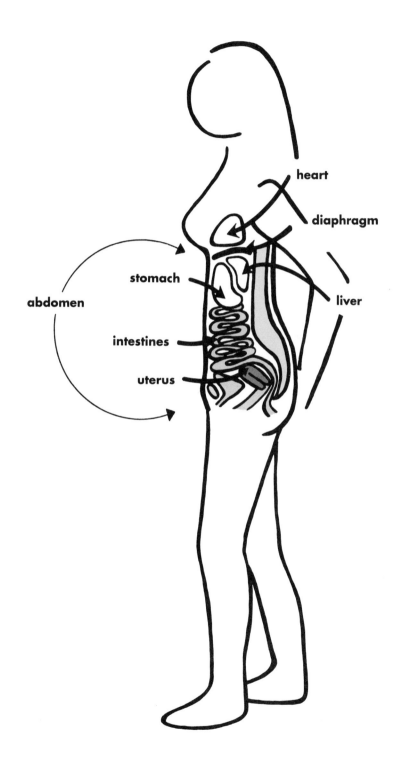

heart

diaphragm

stomach

abdomen

liver

intestines

uterus

As the baby grows larger and larger, the stomach, intestines, liver, and other organs are shoved and squished *up* and *back*. They have much less room.

It becomes especially important to:

- **eat smaller meals more frequently**. There is just not enough room for a large meal to digest well.
- **drink plenty of fluids**. (Eight large glasses of water each day is recommended.) This helps keep the food you've eaten moving through your intestines, and helps prevent indigestion and constipation.
- **eat foods high in fiber**, like whole grains (brown rice, whole-grain cereals, pastas, and breads), beans, salads and other vegetables, and raw fruits. These foods absorb water and help keep your stools soft and regular.
- **avoid hard-to-digest foods, like those high in fat**. Fatty and fried foods, pastries, nuts, nut butters, and even red meats may contribute to indigestion during pregnancy, because they take longer to digest.

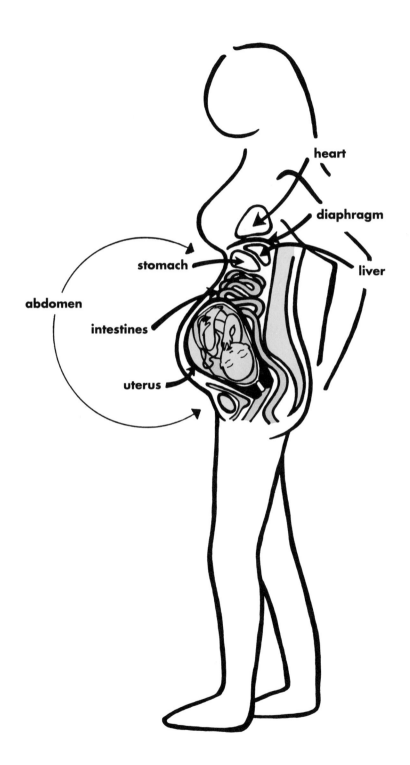

heart

diaphragm

liver

stomach

abdomen

intestines

uterus

THE BLADDER
DURING PREGNANCY

The BLADDER is the small triangle-shaped bag that holds urine. In a woman's body it lies above and behind the *pubic bone* and in front of the *uterus*.

As the baby grows in the *uterus*, the uterus and baby get heavier and heavier, squashing the BLADDER more and more against the pubic bone.

By the 9th month of pregnancy, the BLADDER is squashed completely flat against the pubic bone— usually with the baby's head on one side, and the pubic bone on the other.

BEFORE PREGNANCY

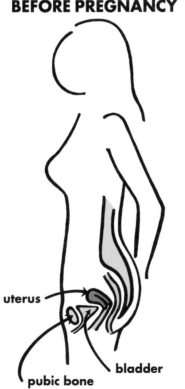

uterus

bladder

pubic bone

This produces a terrific "pressure *on* the bladder"—which feels just like pressure *in* the BLADDER. In other words, the weight of the baby on the BLADDER makes a woman feel like she must urinate. But when she goes to the toilet, only a few drops come out.

She feels the weight of the baby pressing the BLADDER against the pubic bone—which feels just like a full BLADDER.

And whenever she walks or runs, the baby bounces again and again against her BLADDER, usually making her head for the toilet.

9 MONTHS PREGNANT

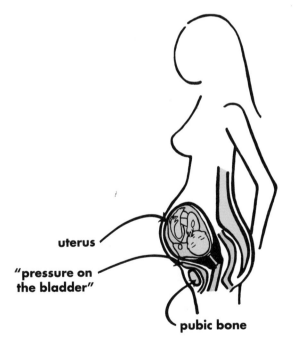

uterus

"pressure on the bladder"

pubic bone

THE MUSCLE OF THE PELVIC FLOOR
(THE "P.C." MUSCLE)

The P.C. muscle extends from the pubic bone in front, to the tail bone or coccyx in back. These two bones give the muscle its full name, the pubococcygeus, or P.C. for short. It has also been called the Kegel muscle, after Dr. Arnold Kegel, who carried out much research into its function.

BLADDER CONTROL

The P.C. muscle is shaped like a hammock and forms the floor of the pelvis. In women it provides support for the bladder, uterus, vagina, and rectum. A strong P.C. muscle ensures good bladder and bowel control. Passing urine when coughing, laughing, sneezing, hiccupping, or burping is a sign of a weak P.C. muscle.

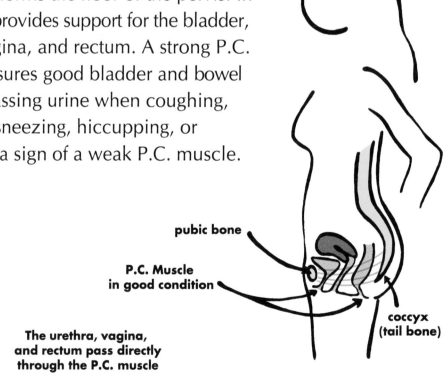

pubic bone

P.C. Muscle
in good condition

coccyx
(tail bone)

The urethra, vagina,
and rectum pass directly
through the P.C. muscle

A strong P.C. muscle keeps you from urinating or moving your bowels at inappropriate moments. Poor P.C. muscle tone leads to incontinence (lack of bladder or bowel control).

A weak muscle cannot support the organs of the pelvic area. The uterus can sag and the urethra and rectum lose support.

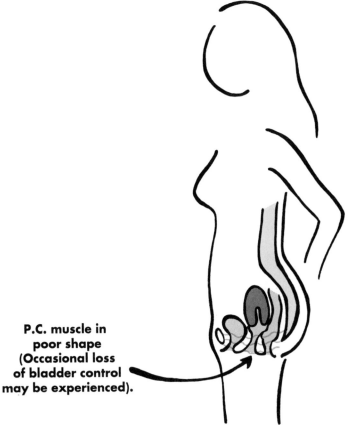

P.C. muscle in poor shape (Occasional loss of bladder control may be experienced).

THE P.C. MUSCLE IN PREGNANCY

Pregnancy puts a lot of pressure on the P.C. muscle, which helps to support the growing uterus and baby, and controls the increased output of urine associated with pregnancy.

During the birth of the child, the P.C. muscle, which surrounds the vagina, gets stretched a great deal by the passage of the baby. Women with a P.C. muscle in good condition experience little difficulty following birth, as the P.C. muscle quickly snaps back into shape. However, women with a weak P.C. muscle may experience a moderate to severe loss of bladder control following birth.

Fortunately, regular exercise of the P.C. muscle during pregnancy can help to ensure good bladder control both during pregnancy and after giving birth.

P.C. muscle in good shape during pregnancy.

HOW TO EXERCISE THE P.C. MUSCLE

The P.C. muscle is exercised by tightening up as if to prevent urination, slowly counting to five, and then relaxing. It can be learned while sitting on the toilet and repeatedly stopping and starting one's flow of urine.

After getting accustomed to the exercise, it can be done anywhere, anytime (while walking, driving, cooking, standing in lines, and so forth. No one will know you are doing it!)

The exercise should be repeated in sets of five or ten at a time throughout the day. During pregnancy it is wise to do between 10 and 20 sets of these *each day*.

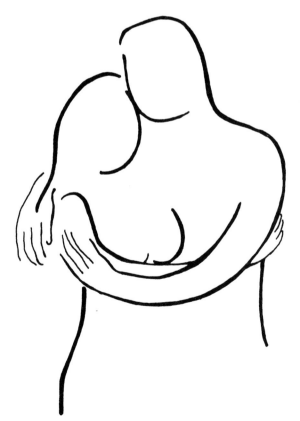

SEXUAL RESPONSE

Women who develop a strong P.C. muscle may discover a marked improvement in their own and their partner's sexual response. A strong P.C. muscle results in a naturally tighter vagina, leading to increased stimulation during intercourse for both partners. Thus, an improved sex life is a happy bonus to the regular exercise of the P.C. muscle.

The amount of blood in a woman's body increases during pregnancy as much as 40%. This is natural and normal, but what does it do to her body?

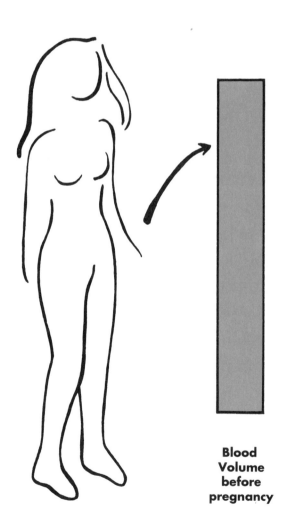
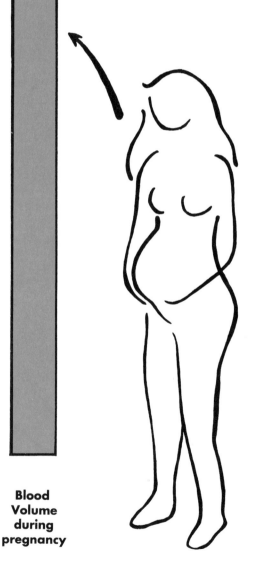

Blood Volume before pregnancy

Blood Volume during pregnancy

VARICOSE VEINS, HEMORRHOIDS, AND FATIGUE

The extra blood volume can cause her blood vessels to swell up. Circulation (movement of the blood) can slow down. Varicose veins (swollen veins) may appear in her legs, she may get hemorrhoids (swollen veins in the rectum), and she may feel tired much of the time.

EXERCISE

At least 20 minutes of low intensity aerobic exercise every day during pregnancy causes her body to produce *more blood vessels, more channels through which the blood can flow*! This reduces swelling in her veins, improves circulation, and she will generally experience an increase in her energy level.

Aerobic exercises are those that are steady and non-stop, and cause an increase in your heart rate. Good aerobic exercises during pregnancy include brisk walking, swimming, and outdoor or stationary bicycling. Running and jogging should generally be avoided as well as any exercise that causes bouncing or jarring of the body, or excessive fatigue. It is also important to wear light clothing and avoid overheating your body when exercising during pregnancy.

It is wise to check with your doctor before beginning any program of exercise while pregnant. Discontinue any exercise that causes vaginal bleeding, spotting, or cramping, and report any such symptoms immediately to your doctor.

POSITION FOR SLEEPING

When a woman is pregnant and sleeps or lies flat on her back, the weight of the baby, and the uterus, and the waters puts pressure on a major body vein (vena cava). This slows down the flow of blood throughout the entire body, and can contribute to abnormal swelling of the legs (edema) and varicose veins. LABOR IS SLOWED DOWN IN THIS POSITION.

A woman with a very large baby or twins can pass out if made to lie on her back. If the circulation of blood throughout the body is slowed down, you will feel tired, even after sleeping.

WRONG POSITION

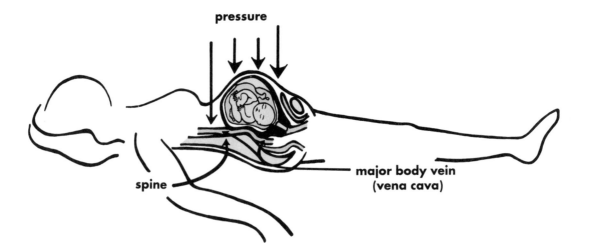

ANY SIDE POSITION IS O.K. FOR SLEEPING OR
RESTING and will help promote good circulation.

RIGHT POSITION

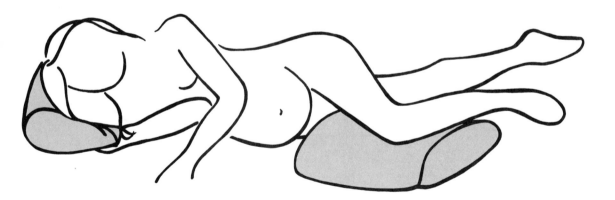

Some people believe that the baby will take whatever it needs from the mother's body. This is just not true! **The foods a pregnant woman eats every day are the foods that build the baby's body.**

The special nutritional needs of the growing baby make it particularly important that the mother's diet be excellent. Through her diet and the care she takes, she gives the child the gift of a poorly or well-formed body.

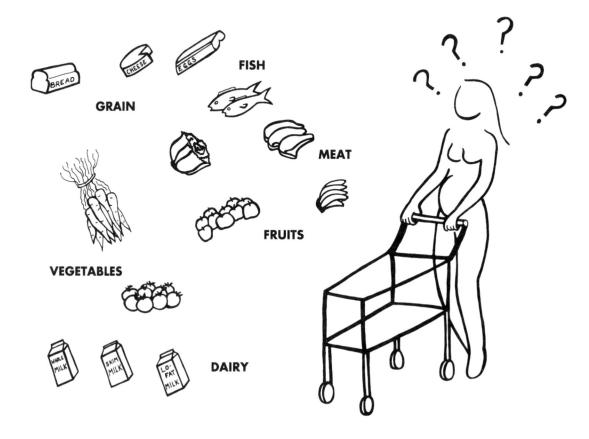

GRAIN

FISH

MEAT

FRUITS

VEGETABLES

DAIRY

hot dog

soda pop

JUNK FOODS CANNOT BUILD A
HEALTHY BODY FOR THE BABY

A POOR DIET DURING
PREGNANCY CAN HELP
CAUSE **BIRTH DEFECTS**.

A GOOD DIET DURING
PREGNANCY CAN HELP ENSURE:
- A normal, healthy, strong baby
- An easy, comfortable pregnancy
- An easier labor and birth
- A healthy, happy mother

ALMOST EVERY COMPLAINT OF
PREGNANCY CAN BE RESOLVED
THROUGH A GOOD DIET AND
PROPER EXERCISE
Many complaints disappear suddenly
as soon as the diet is improved.

WHAT TO EAT

(See worksheet on page 119.)

A well-balanced diet means eating a good variety of foods, like fruits, vegetables, and grains, as well as dairy products (milk and cheeses) and protein foods (meats, fish, eggs, nuts, or beans). It is important to eat foods from each of these groups every day to ensure that the baby gets all the nutrients it needs for a healthy, well-formed body.

Foods lose many important nutrients when they are processed. For instance, a potato contains more food value than potato chips; brown rice contains more food value than white rice or puffed rice; whole wheat flour and whole wheat bread contain more food value than white flour and white bread. Highly processed foods should be avoided. Simply prepared foods provide the most food value.

SWEETS AND FATS

Sweets, like candies, cookies, cakes, and pastries, and *fats*, like butter, lard, cream, and cooking oils, make a pregnant woman feel full, but do not provide much food value for the developing child (or for mom, either). These foods should be avoided or kept to a minimum during pregnancy.

WEIGHT GAIN

The average healthy woman on a good diet during pregnancy gains about 35 pounds. However, if a pregnant woman gains the same amount of weight on *junk* foods, she can really be in trouble. The important thing is not how much weight is gained, but *what kinds* of food she is eating to gain it.

healthy sandwich on whole wheat bread

milk

THE LIVER DURING PREGNANCY

The liver is an organ in your body that helps to clean wastes and some poisons out of your blood. Red blood cells are always being made within your body. They live for about 120 days, and then they die. New red blood cells are always being made to take their place.

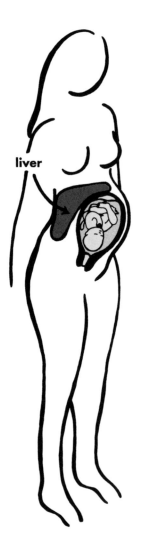

liver

The liver collects up all the dead red blood cells as well as any bits of strange chemicals or poisons you may have eaten, such as the chemical preservatives in some foods, and disposes of them, so your blood can stay clean and healthy. Your liver is working all the time to keep your blood clean.

During pregnancy, the baby's liver is still developing. It does not yet work very well. **Think of the number of times you have to change a baby's diaper after it is born! During pregnancy, all the baby's wastes get dumped into the mother's bloodstream every day, instead**. A pregnant woman's liver must work super hard to help keep her blood clean throughout pregnancy.

Drugs and alcohol are substances your liver works hard to clean out of your body. A pregnant woman's liver is *already* working so hard because of the pregnancy that drugs or alcohol may just be too much. Her overworked liver may not be able to clean the drugs or alcohol out of her blood as fast or as well as it could before pregnancy. Because of this, drugs and alcohol may have a greater effect on a woman during pregnancy. The effect on each woman is different.

Drugs and alcohol taken by a woman during pregnancy go straight to the baby. The problems are first, that **the baby's developing liver cannot easily get these substances out of the baby's body, so they tend to collect in the baby's body in *greater concentrations* than they can be found in the mother's body.** And second, **drugs and alcohol can interfere with the development of the baby's body during pregnancy.**

Drugs and alcohol used by a woman during pregnancy can cause or contribute to a wide variety of birth defects in the child. These substances should be carefully avoided during pregnancy. When medications are necessary during pregnancy, their benefits should be carefully weighed against the possible effect they could have on the unborn child. Alternative measures should be used, whenever possible.

PREVENT BIRTH DEFECTS

The March of Dimes reports that in 1988, one out of every 14 babies born in the U.S. was born with a birth defect. **You can eliminate risks for your child by avoiding the following during pregnancy:**

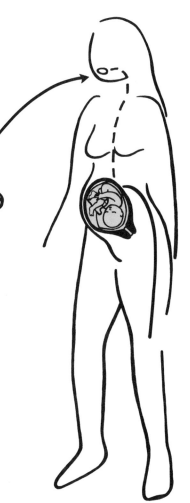

Any drug taken during pregnancy . . . . . . may be harmful to the baby.

(1) Drugs, including non-prescription, over-the-counter medications, or home remedies, like baking soda in water. Many prescription drugs, including sedatives and tranquilizers, have been found to be unsafe during pregnancy.

(2) Smoking cigarettes, or anything at all. Tobacco in all forms.

(3) Alcohol, including beer and wine. There is NO safe level for alcohol consumption during pregnancy.

(4) Illegal drugs, such as marijuana, cocaine, crack, heroin, and PCP have each been shown to create serious health risks for both the pregnant woman and her unborn child.

(5) Coffee, tea, or anything containing caffeine (including cola drinks and chocolate).

(6) Poor nutrition.

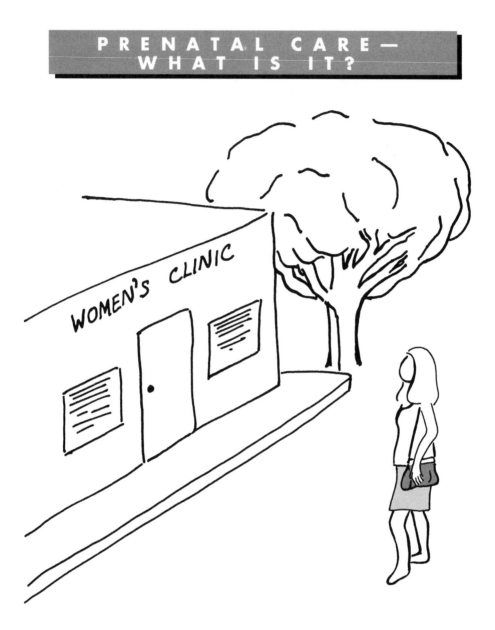

Prenatal care means regular visits to a doctor, midwife, or clinic throughout pregnancy. The schedule of your visits will vary, depending on your practitioner, but usually include:

—an overall physical exam;

This exam should be done early in pregnancy, usually within a week or two of discovering you're pregnant. Your practitioner will confirm your pregnancy, determine the state of your health, and discover any possible problems that need correction—or watching.

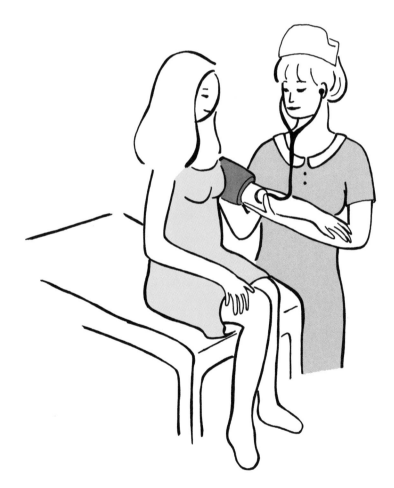

—regular monthly check-ups, up to the 7th month;

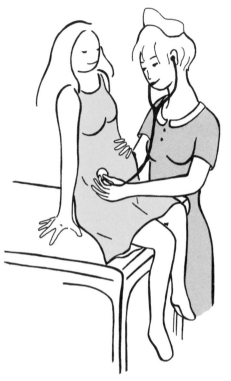

Your doctor or midwife will listen to the baby's heartbeat and measure your uterus (from the outside) to check that your baby is growing normally. He or she will check that you are gaining enough weight, and will also check your blood pressure, and samples of your blood (for anemia) and urine (for sugar and protein). Your doctor or midwife will examine your hands and feet for signs of abnormal swelling (edema). He or she will also discuss any physical problems you may have been having, and try to answer your questions. (Be sure to write down any questions you may have before your check-up.)

—regular check-ups every 2 weeks in the 8th month, and once a week in the 9th month, until the baby is born.

Check-ups will be the same except that now your practitioner will be carefully examining the size and position of the baby, and your cervix (see page 40) to see if it is softening up or thinning out. Your cervix is hard and firm during pregnancy, but softens up just before the baby is ready to be born. Some practitioners speak of the cervix as "green" when it is firm, and "ripe" when it is soft. A soft, "ripe" cervix means the baby will soon be born!

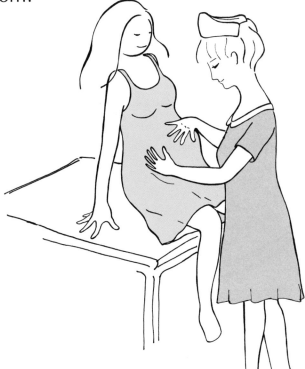

PRENATAL CARE IS IMPORTANT

Through regular prenatal check-ups your doctor or midwife can discover and correct or prevent such problems as *anemia* (low levels of iron and oxygen in your blood), *gestational diabetes* (diabetes which only occurs during pregnancy), and *pre-eclampsia* (a potentially dangerous condition signaled by high blood pressure, abnormal swelling, and protein in the urine). These and other conditions are often *easily corrected when discovered early in pregnancy*, but, if left untreated, can seriously threaten your own health as well as the health and even the life of your baby.

Regular prenatal check-ups, beginning early in pregnancy, help safeguard your own health, and the health and well-being of your baby.

LABOR—WHAT IS IT?

The UTERUS, the large muscle-bag that holds the baby, is the thickest at the CERVIX (opening of the UTERUS) during pregnancy, to safely hold the baby in.

In order for the baby to *come out*, the thick CERVIX becomes thin and then opens wide enough for the baby to pass through.

This thinning (also called effacing) and opening of the CERVIX (dilation) occurs very gradually, little-by-little over a number of hours.

The UTERUS tightens, pulling the CERVIX back just a little, and then relaxes. The tightenings and relaxings of the UTERUS are **CONTRACTIONS OF LABOR**. The CONTRACTIONS continue until the CERVIX is made thin and then pulled open wide enough so the baby can pass through.

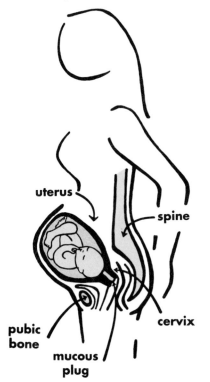

uterus

spine

pubic bone

cervix

mucous plug

**BEFORE LABOR BEGINS.
CERVIX IS THICK.**

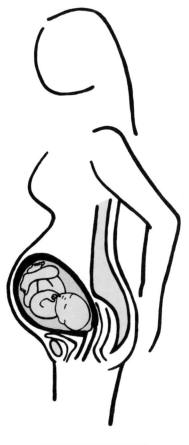

The whole UTERUS, being a muscle, simply rearranges itself. It becomes thin and wide-open at the CERVIX, and thick at the other end. This is all there is to 90% of LABOR. This is the long 1ST STAGE OF LABOR, the rearranging of the UTERUS as it pulls the CERVIX open.

**CERVIX THINNING
BUT NOT OPEN VERY
MUCH. MUCOUS
PLUG IS GONE.**

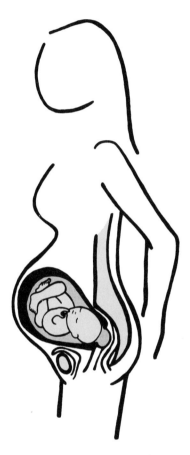

CERVIX HALF-WAY OPEN.

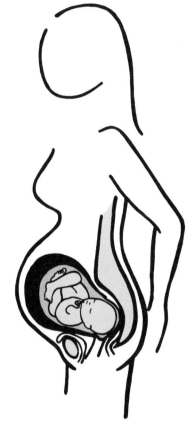

CERVIX FULLY OPEN. "READY TO PUSH BABY OUT."

All that's left is for PUSHING CONTRACTIONS to begin and the thick bottom end of the UTERUS to begin pushing out the baby. (The short 2ND STAGE OF LABOR.)

3 SIGNS OF LABOR

1 **Loss of the mucous plug**. Also called the "bloody show."

As the cervix begins to thin out (efface) and open up (dilate)—the mucous plug falls away, through the vagina, and out of the body. Sometimes small bits of the inside of the cervix are pulled away with it, so there may be blood with the mucous plug, from the inside edges of the cervix, to which it was attached. When this happens, the loss of the mucous plug is called the "bloody show." (There is no pain or discomfort associated with the loss of the mucous plug or "bloody show.")

The loss of the mucous plug or "bloody show" is a sign that the cervix has begun to thin out (efface) and open up (dilate). So, it is a sign that *labor* has begun.

FALSE LABOR

Many women have "false labor" or many little practice contractions during the last month or two of pregnancy.

These small "practice" contractions are not real labor because the baby is not yet ready to be born. But, they can cause the cervix to thin out (efface) and even open up (dilate) a little, as much as a month or more before real labor begins.

And so sometimes the mucous plug is lost—or the "bloody show" is seen weeks before real labor begins. If this happens, it usually means real labor will be shorter than average, and is nothing to worry about. Your doctor should be informed, however, any time this sign of labor is seen.

NOTE: The mucous plug is often lost without it being noticed, during one of a pregnant woman's frequent trips to the toilet.

2 Contractions. (Tightening and relaxing of the uterus as it works to open up (dilate) the cervix.)

This is the surest sign that labor has begun—regular contractions that do not go away no matter what a woman is doing and no matter what position she is in.

Because "practice" contractions (false labor) are common, the best way to tell if these contractions are really labor is to walk around, take a warm shower, or otherwise change your position and activity. If the contractions turn off, it was probably "false labor."

But, if the contractions do not turn off but get stronger and closer together after changing your activity and position several times, then you are probably in labor for sure!

If you also pass blood or mucous from the vagina at this time, you can be sure you are in real labor.

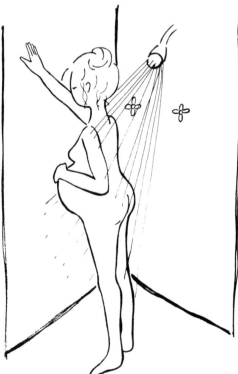

3 Amnion (Bag-of-Waters) Breaks. If the amnion (bag-of-waters) breaks at any time during pregnancy, a woman should always call her doctor or midwife to let him or her know. Contractions should begin within 12 to 24 hours from the time the amnion (bag-of-waters) breaks. Contractions may also begin immediately.

It is wise to put a rubber sheet over your mattress, under your regular sheet, to protect the mattress in case the amnion (bag-of-waters) breaks while you're in bed.

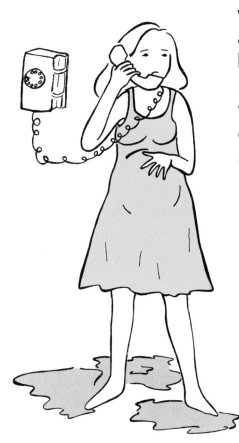

About 30% of all women with good nutrition have the amnion (bag-of-waters) break as their first sign of labor. Almost all women who have had *poor nutrition* during pregnancy have the amnion (bag-of-waters) break as their first sign of labor.

THE PURPOSE OF CONTRACTIONS

1st Stage Labor

The whole *purpose* of contractions is to *dilate the cervix, to pull it* open so that the baby can come out. For this reason, a woman should consciously RELAX her vaginal area and the rest of her body every time she has a contraction, to help the cervix to open (dilate) as wide as it can.

REST PERIODS

Remember, contractions of labor turn on and *off.* They allow a woman to *rest* between them. Contractions every 4 minutes mean only 15 contractions in an hour. And the closer together (and stronger!) the contractions are, the sooner the baby will be born!

Contractions of labor accelerate or speed up, much as a car gathers speed as you shift into higher gears. When contractions begin, they usually only last 30 seconds, and may be 20 minutes or more apart.

Gradually, the contractions get closer together—15 minutes apart, 10 minutes apart, 5 minutes apart—3 minutes apart.

Gradually, little by little, the contractions get longer—30 seconds long, 45 seconds long, 1 minute long, 1 1/2 minutes long. Sometimes, just before it's time to push out the baby, contractions may even be lasting 2 minutes!

The *stronger* and *closer together* the contractions get, *the faster the cervix is opening.*

DILATION OF THE CERVIX

Drawings are actual size

The WORK of real labor is in *relaxing* the rest of your body *completely* while the *uterus* is working harder and faster to open the *cervix*. And it is **work**. It can take anywhere from 2 to 24 hours, or more, for the cervix of a normal healthy woman to open fully so that she is ready to push out the baby.

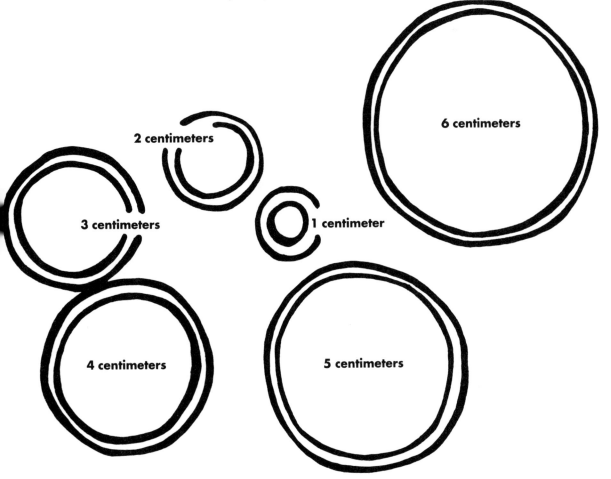

2 centimeters

6 centimeters

3 centimeters

1 centimeter

4 centimeters

5 centimeters

As soon as the cervix is open fully (to 10 centimeters) the contractions ease up. They get *shorter, farther apart*, and *less strong*. This is always a very welcome break from the very strong, very long and close-together contractions that come just before full dilation.

As soon as the cervix is open fully (to 10 centimeters) a woman gets to push out her baby. This is usually the most fun and exciting part for everyone!

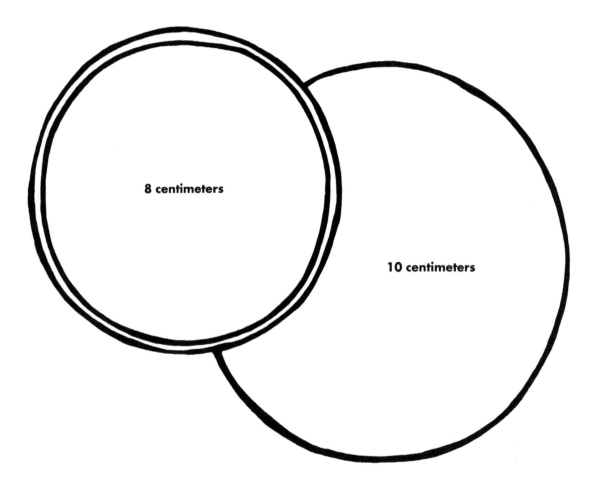

VAGINAL EXAMS DURING
1ST STAGE LABOR

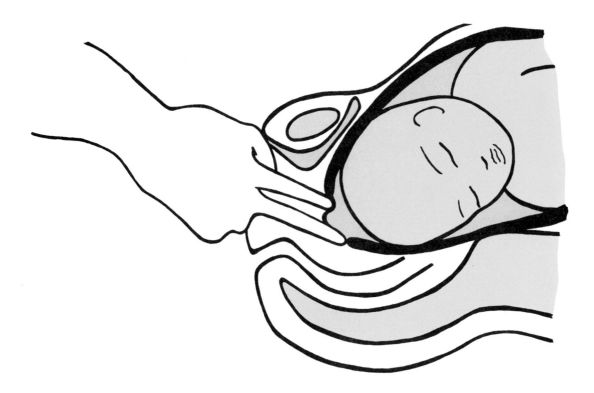

Doctor, nurse, or midwife's hand is shown checking how far the cervix has opened (dilated). The woman in labor is on her back—just for the *vaginal exam*.

The cervix has opened (dilated) to about 3 centimeters. The amnion (bag-of-waters) has not yet broken.

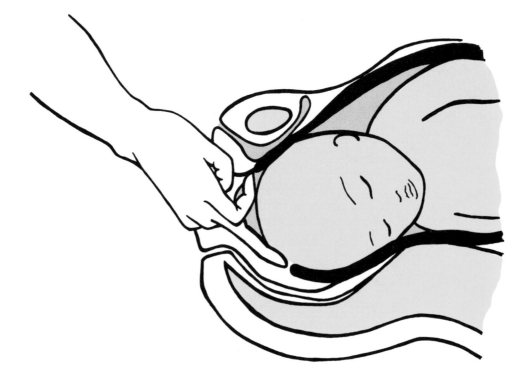

The cervix has opened (dilated) to about 7 or 8 centimeters. The amnion (bag-of-waters) has not yet broken. The baby has moved down and the bladder and rectum are under a lot of pressure.

The cervix is fully open. (Dilated to 10 centimeters.) The baby's head has come *through* the cervix.

The amnion (bag-of-waters) has not yet broken. The rectum is squeezed flat against the bottom of the spine, and the bladder is under a lot more pressure too.

Now she's ready to *push out the baby!*

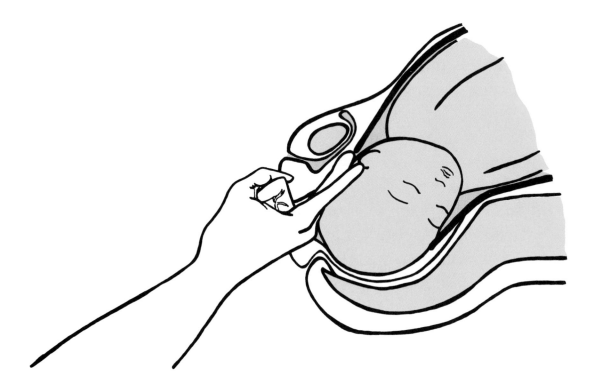

TRANSITION

The word *transition* means *a period of change.*
Transition in labor means the change in the action of
the uterus, from *opening up* the cervix (the long 1st
stage of labor, dilation) to *pushing out the baby* (the
short 2nd stage of labor).

This is a major change for the woman's body and
the blood circulation undergoes a major change. The
blood concentrates in the area of the uterus.

Transition can be called the last 2 or 3 centimeters
of dilation—or when the cervix goes from 7 to 10
centimeters—and includes the whole time it takes for
the contractions to change over from *opening
contractions* to *pushing contractions.*

Transition is the shortest and least comfortable part
of labor. It lasts between 10 minutes and an hour. One
half hour is about the average length of transition.

TRANSITION is the change from

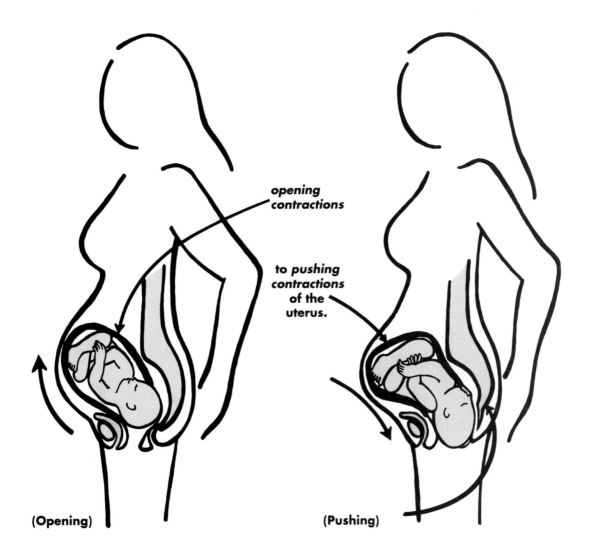

opening contractions

to pushing contractions of the uterus.

(Opening)

(Pushing)

The lower part of the spine (tail bone or coccyx) becomes flexible and can straighten out, making more room for the baby as it passes through the birth canal and out into the world.

SIGNS OF TRANSITION

It is important to recognize the signs of transition *because these signs tell you it's almost time to push out the baby*! No woman has *all* these signs of transition but most women have two or three of them.

Legs or body trembling (caused by circulation changes)

Hot or cold flashes (also caused by circulation changes)

Feeling like having to have a bowel movement (pressure of the baby as it moves down, pressing the rectum against the bottom of the spine)

Nausea or vomiting (depends on what you last ate, and when it was)

Burping

Hiccupping

Confusion

Bad disposition—mother may feel irritable

Feeling of wanting to leave (wherever you are)

Strongest contractions (contractions may become very painful)

Longest contractions

Contractions closest together (may be as close as 20 seconds apart)

An understanding Coach is the *most* help during transition. Back rubs or pressure may feel good.

Remember, transition is a *very short* period. As soon as 2nd Stage Labor begins and the woman starts to *push out the baby*, **the signs of transition disappear**. The excitement and work of pushing out the baby takes over.

The BIRTH of the baby—*pushing out the baby*—is called 2nd Stage Labor. It is much shorter than 1st Stage Labor (dilation). 2nd Stage Labor (pushing out the baby) can take 20 minutes or less, or an hour or more. But it *rarely* takes longer than 2 hours.

Pushing is hard work, most of the time. But pushing in 2nd Stage Labor is a different kind of work from the work of relaxing through contractions in 1st Stage Labor.

Pushing out a baby is not painful at all to most women. But there is a *lot of pressure* as the baby moves down and out. Some women are surprised to discover pleasurable sensations in 2nd Stage Labor.

And pushing out a baby is *always* exciting and a terrific emotional thrill.

In pushing, the *uterus* works automatically and pushes every time it contracts. But *a woman pushes with her abdominal muscles* to help the uterus. The push of the uterus is automatic; the push of the abdominal muscles is done by the woman. It usually takes both muscles working to push out a baby.

2ND STAGE LABOR

Pushing out the Baby

Mother is usually supported by her coach,
or many pillows, while pushing. Adjustable
beds or delivery tables make pushing
(2nd Stage Labor) easier.

Effective position for pushing
—*modified squatting position.*

A woman helps the uterus by pushing with her abdominal (stomach) muscles.

The uterus pushes automatically, all by itself.

It usually takes both the uterus *and* the woman pushing with her abdominal (stomach) muscles, in order to *push out a baby*.

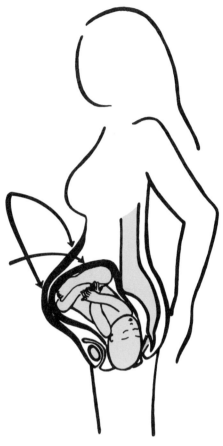

While both the uterus and the abdominal muscles are working to push out the baby, the baby moves some distance down the birth canal. Between contractions, when both muscles are relaxed, the baby usually slips back a little. Pushing is a 2 down, 1 back, 2 down, 1 back kind of thing—until the baby's head starts to crown (the baby's head is seen in the vaginal opening, with the vaginal opening forming a "crown" around the baby's head). Then the baby stays right there and doesn't slip back anymore.

Next—the baby is *out*!

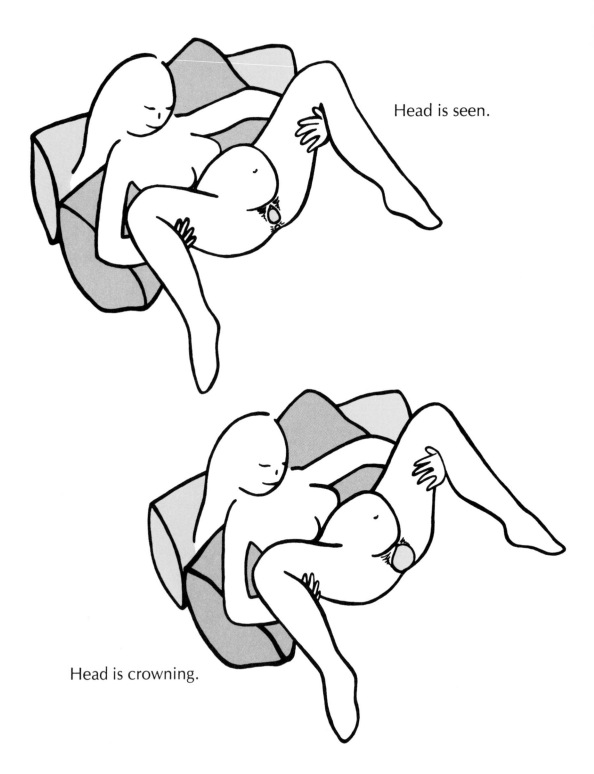

Head is seen.

Head is crowning.

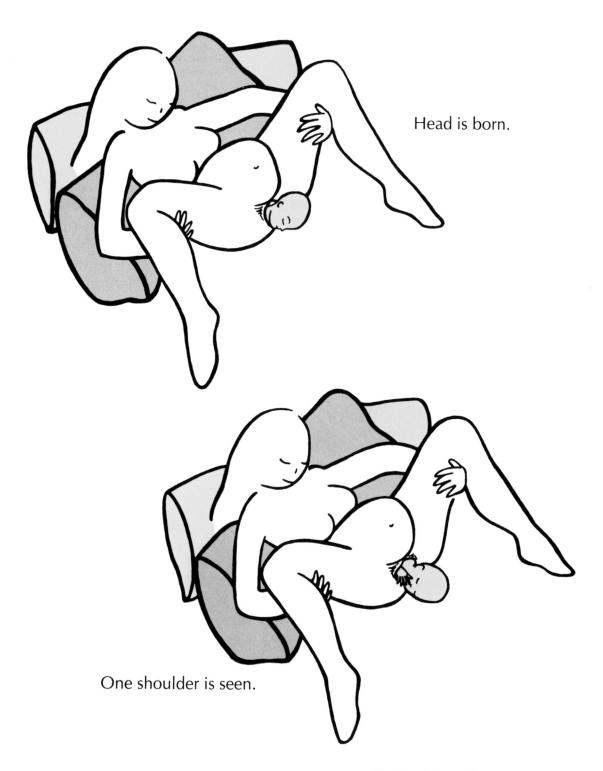

Head is born.

One shoulder is seen.

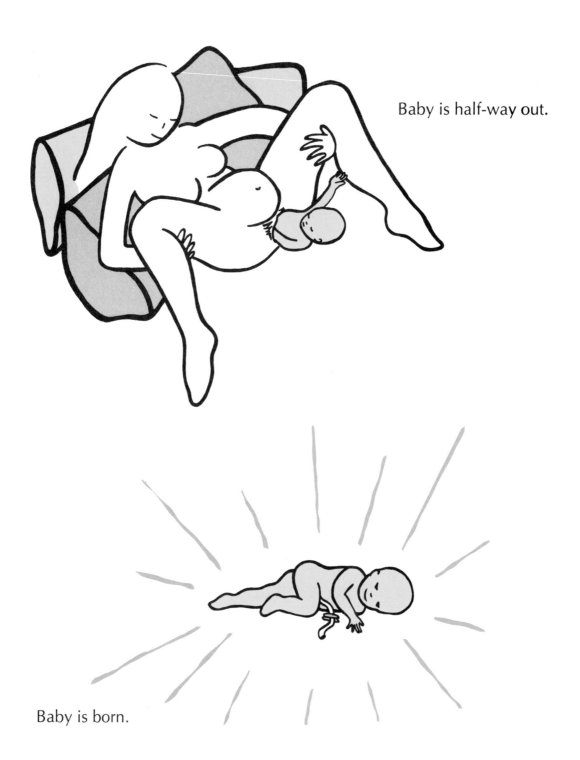

Baby is half-way out.

Baby is born.

Pushing out the "Afterbirth"

3rd Stage is the last stage of labor. It is the shortest stage of labor and usually takes less than 15 minutes. The placenta is separating from the inside of the uterus.

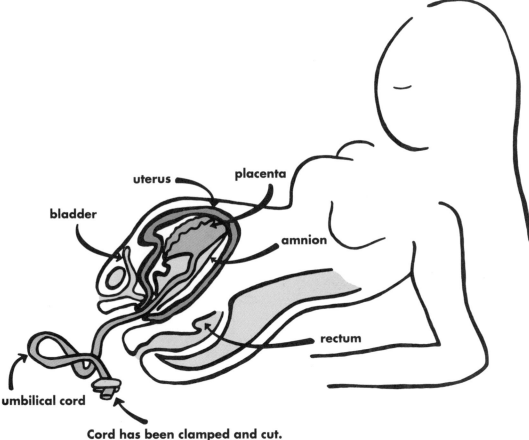

uterus

placenta

bladder

amnion

rectum

umbilical cord

Cord has been clamped and cut.

The placenta separating from the inside of the uterus.

All that happens in 3rd Stage Labor is the woman pushes out the *afterbirth* (placenta, umbilical cord, and amnion). She will feel the uterus contract several more times—and she pushes with the uterus, using her abdominal muscles, just as she did in 2nd Stage Labor when she pushed out the *baby*. (Except that pushing out the afterbirth is *much easier* than pushing out the baby.)

THE "AFTERBIRTH"

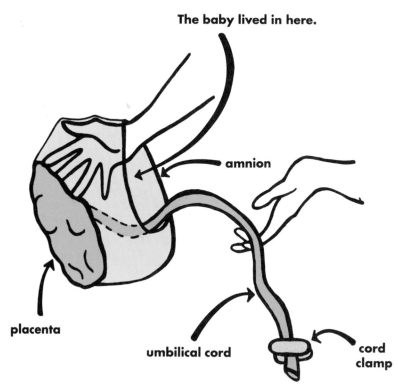

The baby lived in here.

amnion

placenta

umbilical cord

cord clamp

The bladder and rectum have been stretched out of shape by the birth of the child.

The large uterus sags. It is empty now that the afterbirth has been pushed out.

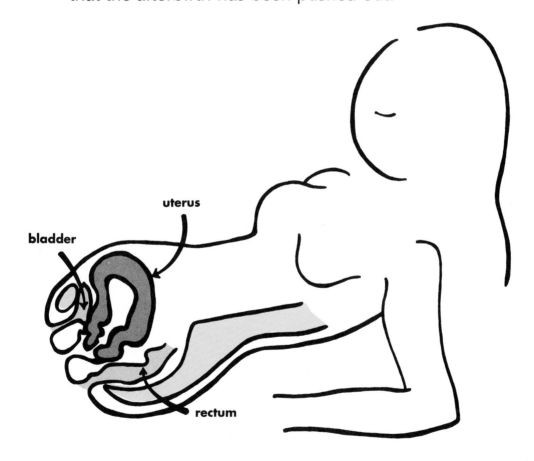

bladder

uterus

rectum

MASSAGE THE "FUNDUS"

The part of the uterus where the placenta was attached is full of open blood vessels, and will be bleeding freely after the placenta separates from the uterus.

In order to keep the new mother from bleeding too much, the *fundus* of the uterus (that part of the uterus farthest from the opening) is massaged or rubbed gently by the mother or coach, beginning as soon as the afterbirth comes out.

The massage or *gentle* rub of the fundus makes the uterus *contract*. This cuts down on the bleeding as the insides of the uterus press against themselves.

HOW TO MASSAGE THE FUNDUS

One just *gently* rubs the whole lower abdomen, below the navel. When something gets hard, continue to rub that, it's the *fundus*. It should be kept "hard as a billiard ball and below the navel" for the first day after the baby is born. Rub the fundus about every 15 minutes.

Between massages the uterus will relax and spread out, but it should be kept contracted into a hard ball, and *below the navel*. This helps to keep the new mother from bleeding too much after the baby is born.

RUB GENTLY every 15 minutes the 1st day.

fundus:
Keep it "hard as a billiard ball and below the navel."

uterus

INVOLUTION

Involution means the return of an organ (such as the uterus) to its normal size after it has become stretched or enlarged.

It takes about 6 weeks for involution to be completed and the uterus, bladder, and rectum of most women to return to their normal shapes after childbirth. The inside of the uterus, where the placenta was attached, will be healing up. Nothing should enter the vagina until this healing is completed. (About 6 weeks.) Sexual intercourse or use of tampons should be avoided during this time.

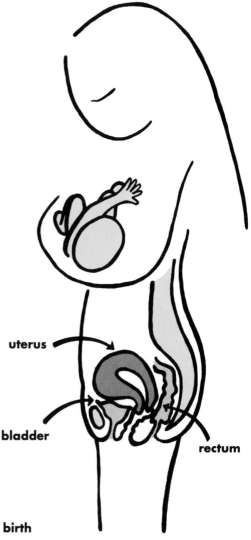

uterus

bladder

rectum

5 days after the birth

BREASTFEEDING

If the new mother *breastfeeds* the baby soon after it is born, and frequently throughout the first few days, a hormone will be released in the mother's body that also helps keep the uterus contracted, protecting the mother from too much bleeding after the birth.

Continuing to breastfeed an infant can help a new mother regain her figure following childbirth. While breastfeeding, new mothers should maintain an excellent, well-balanced diet, so their milk supply can be of consistent high quality.

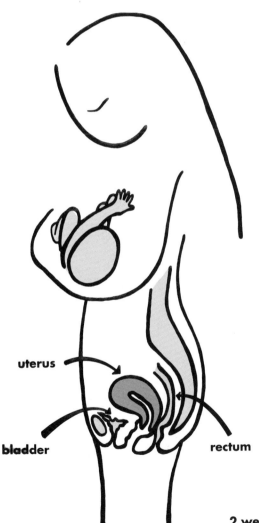

uterus

bladder

rectum

2 weeks after the birth

A new baby needs to be kept warm, to eat, and to sleep. The baby will spend most of the first week sleeping. Most babies will wake to nurse every 2 or 3 hours, nurse for about 30 minutes or so, and then go back to sleep. Very sleepy babies can be gently awakened and encouraged to nurse (in the daytime) if they have slept at least 3 hours. This can help the baby to sleep for longer periods of time at night.

APPEARANCE

Normal newborns may appear a bit wrinkled and puffy-looking after all the squeezing and pushing of labor and birth. Eyes are blue-gray but will change color in the coming months. So will the baby's skin. All newborns, regardless of race, appear pink-skinned at birth. Darker skin pigments take hours or days to develop. The skin of a new baby, especially upon the hands and feet, may seem to be peeling off within the first week or so. This is just a protective coating that covers the baby's skin before birth, becoming dry and rubbing off.

ROOMING IN

After giving birth in a hospital or birth center, it is best for the new mother and baby to stay together at all times. This is called "rooming in" and permits the new mother to breastfeed and to respond directly to her baby's needs. While the new mother gets to know her baby, the baby learns to nurse, to feel secure, and to trust the mother. The newborn can see, hear, smell, taste, and is especially sensitive to touch.

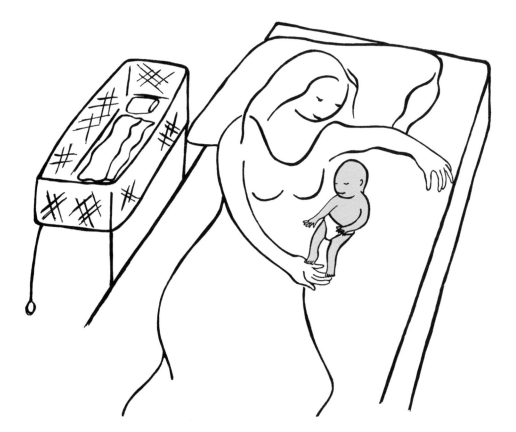

THE CORD

The cord, which has been clamped and cut, should be kept clean and dry. The place where baby and cord meet should be swabbed with alcohol twice a day until the cord becomes completely dry. No oils should be used in this area, and no baths given, until the cord falls off. (The baby can be wiped clean with a damp cloth until then.) The cord will fall off, usually within 7 to 10 days, leaving the navel (belly button).

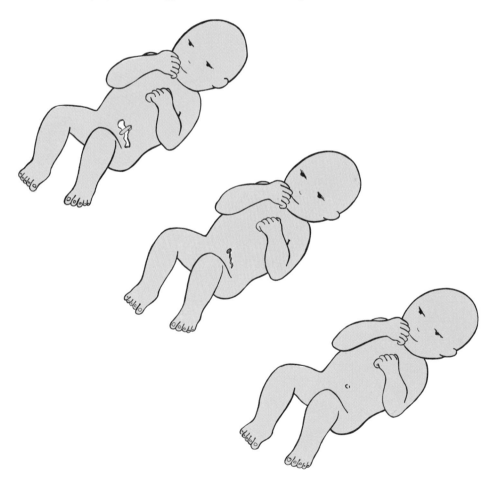

BOWEL MOVEMENTS

The baby's first bowel movements are black and sticky, like thick tar. They stain cloth diapers, no matter how many times you wash or bleach them. The loose, shapeless stools of a breastfed newborn usually appear by the end of the first week.

WEIGHT LOSS

Most babies lose a few ounces the first week. They are usually gaining weight again within 7 to 9 days. Babies whose mothers received anesthetics during labor and birth often suck less vigorously and with less frequency. They tend to lose more weight than natural childbirth babies whose mothers received no birth anesthetic. Breastfeeding a newborn on demand from the day (or hour) of birth minimizes newborn weight loss and helps a new mother's breastmilk "come in."

BREASTFEEDING

True breastmilk doesn't appear within a new mother's breasts for 3 or 4 days. Before that time her breasts contain **colostrum**, which is much higher in protein than breastmilk, and is designed to protect the tiny newborn from disease. Colostrum has been called "**nature's vaccine**" as it begins to protect the baby with the first feeding.

There is nothing a new baby can be fed which is more important to its health and well-being than colostrum. Giving the baby a bottle (of *anything*) within the first few weeks can confuse the baby and create difficulties with breastfeeding. Nursing at the mother's breast is more work than sucking from a bottle. Learning (the easier) task of sucking from a bottle can cause some babies to reject the mother's breast.

JAUNDICE

A new baby's liver is immature and has difficulty cleaning all the waste products from its blood. (During pregnancy, the placenta and the mother's liver performed this function.) When the liver is not efficient in cleaning a newborn's bloodstream, the baby's skin may appear yellow. This is called jaundice.

Almost half of all normal newborns show some signs of jaundice, beginning on the 2nd to the 4th day of life. Usually the jaundice disappears by the end of the first week and causes no problem. However, **jaundice that appears within the first 24 hours or after the first week could be harmful to the baby and should be reported immediately to your doctor.** Similarly, if your baby develops a *deep* yellow color, he or she should be checked by a pediatrician.

THE BABY'S BED

New babies seem to sleep well on a smooth, firm surface. Raising the level of the baby's mattress 2 inches higher at the head than at the foot may protect the baby from potentially harmful breathing problems.

THE FIRST WEEK—THE MOTHER

EMOTIONAL LET-DOWN (BLUES)

After all the months of anticipation and preparation, the baby has arrived. Many mothers are thrilled, but it is not uncommon to feel just the opposite—empty, numb, sad, or a bit "lost." A similar sort of emotional let-down is often experienced after other major life events for which you have planned and prepared. The big day comes, and then it's over. The excitement and anticipation that had filled your days are gone. It is common (and natural) to feel emotionally "let down" or "blue."

The physical demands of recovering from pregnancy and childbirth, as well as those of adjusting to the needs of the baby, provide additional stress. Body image can be another problem. No longer pregnant, many women feel fat. For mothers who breastfeed, the extra pounds usually fall away without too much trouble, but it may be six months or more before the old clothes fit.

GET PLENTY OF REST—DON'T OVEREXERT

New mothers need to take it easy. They need to rest, and to nap when the baby naps. If a new mother tries to do too much too soon, she can suddenly feel very tired, and she may even faint. For the first few weeks after giving birth, plenty of rest is important. **New mothers who are well rested produce better-quality breastmilk, and more of it, than mothers who are anxious.**

Husband, family, or friends can help with house-cleaning, marketing, laundry, cooking, and care of older children during the first few weeks. New mothers do best when all they have to care for is themselves and the new baby. That's plenty!

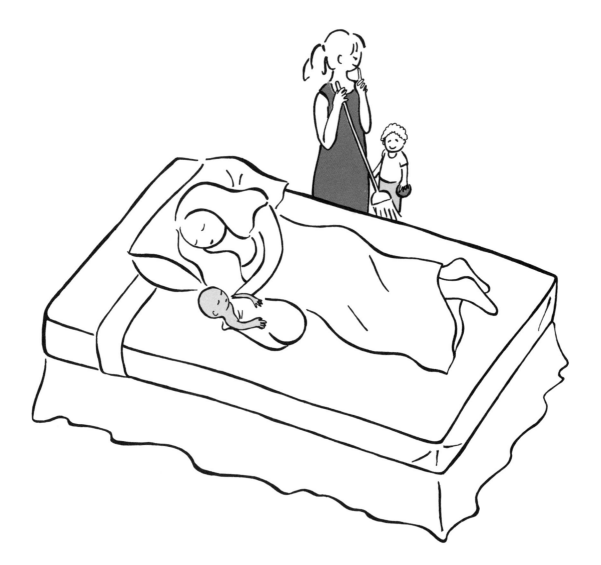

BLEEDING

New mothers can expect vaginal bleeding for 2 to 6 weeks following childbirth (almost as if you'd "saved up" all those menstrual periods you missed). This is normal. It comes from the inside of the uterus where the placenta was attached, and continues until the healing in that area is complete.

Bleeding is usually heaviest the first 3 to 5 days, and clots are not uncommon. The use of hospital-size sanitary napkins and old towels or pads to protect your bed (and the floor beside the bed, since the blood tends to "gush out") when you get up in the morning can help prevent accidental stains or spots.

The blood is bright red for the first few days, becomes watery, then dark-red, brown, and even a bit yellow before it disappears. It may stop and start a few times before it's truly gone.

Sanitary napkins should be used to catch the blood (not tampons), and sexual intercourse should also be avoided, until the uterus is healed and the bleeding has stopped. Inserting anything into the vagina before healing is complete introduces a serious risk of infection for the mother.

Mothers who breastfeed may experience somewhat less bleeding, since breastfeeding causes the uterus to contract and helps the inside of the uterus to heal. Eating plenty of dark green vegetables and salads may speed healing and shorten the bleeding for some women. Vigorous exercise begun within the first 6 weeks can prolong bleeding, or start it up again if it has already stopped.

TROUBLE SIGNS

The following signs should be reported to your doctor. They could mean trouble:

- **Extra-heavy bleeding,** which soaks through more than one large pad an hour, for several hours.
- **Bright red bleeding** after the fourth day, especially if heavy.
- **Foul smelling odor.** After birth bleeding should smell like regular menstrual bleeding. A bad smell is usually a sign of infection.
- **Abdominal cramping** that begins after the fourth day.
- **Unusually large clots.** (Small clots, about half the size of a woman's thumb, are normal.)

SHOWERS ONLY, NO BATHS!

Baths should be avoided until after the bleeding stops, to reduce the risk of infection. *Only showers* or *"sponge baths"* should be taken.

CAUTION. Within the first week new mothers may *faint* in the shower. A husband, family member, or friend should stand by, in the bathroom, the first few times a new mother showers, just in case she suddenly feels faint and needs assistance.

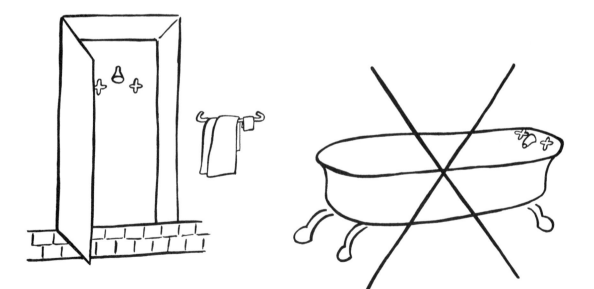

AFTER-BIRTH CONTRACTIONS

Breastfeeding a newborn causes the release of a hormone that makes the uterus contract and helps a new mother get back into shape. Smaller amounts of the same hormone are released when a new mother sees, hears, touches, holds, or even *thinks* about her baby.

First-time mothers usually notice little or no "after-birth contractions." Women who have already had one or more children may experience strong abdominal cramping. These contractions come and go, but can feel as uncomfortable as the contractions of active labor, and may be felt for as long as 4 or 5 days.

Every woman does not experience uncomfortable after-birth contractions, but for those who do, relaxation, slow, deep breathing, and patience are the answer. The after-birth contractions will pass. **ASPIRIN** should *never* be taken for relief of after-birth contraction discomfort because it can lead to dangerous bleeding in new mothers. Other drugs should also be avoided, as they pass directly into the breastmilk and to the baby.

SORE BOTTOM

The birth of a baby causes most new mothers to experience external vaginal swelling and soreness for the first few days, whether or not stitches were required. An ice pack (easily made by soaking a sanitary napkin in water, squeezing out the excess, and freezing it) feels wonderful! A dozen or more can be made so they may be exchanged whenever the coldness wears off.

CARE OF STITCHES

If stitches were used to repair a tear or an incision of the vaginal opening, care must be taken to keep the area clean in order to prevent infection and to promote rapid healing. The stitched area should be washed with a disinfectant (like betadine) after every visit to the toilet. Always wash from front to back. This may sting, but is essential if a painful and troublesome infection is to be avoided. Antiseptic powder may also be applied after the area has been washed with the disinfectant.

FLUIDS

New mothers are advised to drink plenty of fluids—the equivalent of 8 to 10 large glasses of water each day. This helps to replace fluids lost in childbirth, and aids in the production of breastmilk.

CONSTIPATION

If a new mother isn't drinking enough fluids her stools can become rock-hard and dry. It is especially important to keep a new mother's stools soft and regular following childbirth. Hard stools are more difficult for new mothers to pass, and can necessitate such straining that hemorrhoids can result.

Fruits, salads and other vegetables, whole grains, beans, and especially dried fruit (such as apricots or prunes), prune juice, or flax seed (an excellent natural laxative) continue to be important in the diet of a new mother, especially during the first few weeks following the birth of a child.

EXCESSIVE PERSPIRATION

Some new mothers perspire heavily, even while sleeping, almost drenching their sheets and bed clothes. Such perspiration is nature's way of getting rid of the extra fluids so important during pregnancy (for the maintenance of increased blood volume and amniotic fluid) that are no longer needed by the non-pregnant woman. Once the body's normal fluid balance is achieved, the heavy perspiration ends.

FEVER

Though rare, fever occasionally occurs following childbirth. **Any fever that occurs in a woman within the first 2 weeks after childbirth can be dangerous and should be reported immediately to a doctor.**

Some women experience a low fever when their milk "comes in." This passes in a day or two when the nursing relationship becomes established, and is no cause for alarm.

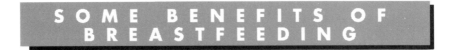
THE BEST FOOD FOR BABIES

Breastmilk provides an infant with complete nutrition. Pediatricians strongly recommend breastfeeding, as overall, breastmilk provides **better nutrition than formulas.** Breastmilk is also **cheaper and easier** than infant formulas. It costs nothing and is **always fresh and ready.**

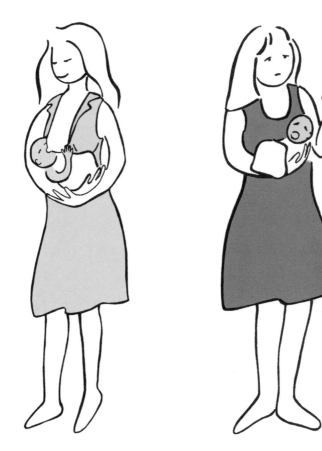

PROTECTION FROM DISEASE

Through breastmilk, babies share in the immunity to diseases their mothers have built up over a lifetime. **Breastfed babies get fewer illnesses** than bottle-fed babies, and the illnesses they do get are generally less severe. Doctors throughout the world are working to promote better health for babies by encouraging mothers to breastfeed **at least throughout the first year of life.** Semi-solids and finger-foods can be added between the 5th and the 8th month, *but not before.* You know a child is ready for these foods when he or she puts everything within reach into his or her mouth!

PROTECTION FROM ALLERGIES

Babies are never allergic to their own mother's milk. Occasionally a baby may react to something specific the mother ate. The answer is simply to eliminate that food from the mother's diet.

Babies **can** develop allergies when other foods are introduced too early, especially formulas based on or containing cow's milk. Cow's milk is the perfect food for a **calf,** but should NOT be fed to human infants, especially during the first twelve months of life. Feeding a baby cow's milk or a formula based on or containing cow's milk can sometimes lead to a lifetime of allergic problems. Breastfeeding may also reduce the chance of a baby developing allergies *later* in life.

EASIER TO DIGEST

Breastmilk is so fully and easily digested that a breastfed baby's stools have **no foul odor.** They are normally quite loose and shapeless, range in color from yellow or mustard to green, and have only a mild smell, which is not at all unpleasant.

Formula preparations are more difficult for a baby to digest. Rather than digesting fully, like breastmilk, part of the formula can spoil within the baby's intestinal system. This produces the strong, foul-smelling odor common to the more solid stools of most bottle-fed babies. This also produces intestinal gas, which can cause painful pressures and a crying, "colicky" baby.

HELPS MOM GET BACK INTO SHAPE

Breastfeeding a baby helps a new mother get back into shape in two ways. First, nursing a baby causes a hormone to be released that helps contract or "shrink" the enlarged uterus. Breastfeeding actually helps pull a new mother's insides back into shape **every time the baby nurses.**

Second, a nursing mother produces many quarts of milk each week. This milk production burns up lots of calories and can make it easier for nursing mothers to lose extra pounds following childbirth.

NATURAL TRANQUILIZER

Hormones released by breastfeeding also work upon the mother as a natural tranquilizer. This helps mothers who breastfeed feel patient, calm, and relaxed as they nurse.

A SPECIAL RELATIONSHIP

Mothers who breastfeed enjoy a special closeness with their babies that is deeply satisfying. Besides all its other benefits, breastfeeding is a lot of fun!

TO LEARN MORE ABOUT BREASTFEEDING

Read **The Womanly Art of Breastfeeding**, by La Leche League International, or contact a La Leche League group. La Leche is Spanish and means "the milk." La Leche League is a non-profit organization formed in 1956 by seven women to provide information and encouragement to breastfeeding mothers. It has become a highly respected worldwide organization with over 3,000 La Leche League groups in 44 countries.

To find the La Leche League group nearest you, call your local library, the maternity department of your largest hospital, or an obstetrician or pediatrician. Or you can contact La Leche League at its headquarters in Franklin Park, Illinois. If you send them a self-addressed, stamped envelope, they will send you a list of the La Leche League groups and leaders nearest you at no charge. Contact: **La Leche League International, 9616 Minneapolis Ave., P.O. Box 1209, Franklin Park, Illinois 60131-8209**. Or call **(708) 455-7730** between 9 A.M. and 3 P.M. central time. At other times a prerecorded message will refer you to another number for immediate breastfeeding help.

CHILDBIRTH CLASSES

Pregnancy, birth and parenting a child or children—what an amazing adventure it is! Few, if any, of the things we do are quite as important or mean so much to us. Yet *most* of us are not very well prepared for *any* of these jobs.

If you are expecting a child, search out good childbirth classes in your area. They are a fun way to prepare, both physically and emotionally, for the birth of your child. And they can make an enormous difference in your birth experience. Women and men who attend childbirth classes tend to enjoy the birth process more than those who do not.

It has also been shown that attending childbirth classes can reduce the incidence of complications of pregnancy and birth for *both mother and child.*

(1) **Eat a wide variety of foods.** This will help to ensure that the baby gets all the necessary ingredients for a strong, well-formed body.

(2) **Avoid added sugars.** Eliminate table sugar, syrups, and sweets. If sugar or syrup is one of the first four ingredients listed on a package, *don't buy it!* These refined sugars provide empty calories. They can make you feel full without providing good nutrition for the baby. And they can help you gain unnecessary weight.

(3) **Avoid fatty or fried foods.** These are hard to digest, and can contribute to heartburn or indigestion. Pork and lamb take longer to digest than other meats and should probably be eaten sparingly or avoided during pregnancy, too.

(4) **Eat whole grains only.** This includes breads, cereals, rice, pastas, and tortillas. These products made with the complete whole grain provide more food value for the baby and valuable fiber to help prevent constipation. Learn to read the labels on packages before purchasing your food, as some breads made with white, refined grains contain food coloring to make them look like the healthier whole-grain version.

(5) **Eat smaller meals more frequently.** Women who skip meals during pregnancy can faint suddenly, which can be dangerous for both mother and child.

During pregnancy, your stomach and intestines get shoved and squished up and back by the growing uterus and baby. You no longer have room to handle a large meal. Smaller meals, eaten more frequently, will be far more comfortable, and are digested more easily.

Nausea, a common complaint of pregnancy, can often be prevented by nibbling or "grazing" throughout the day. Morning sickness (nausea in the morning) can sometimes be prevented by eating a little snack in the middle of the night, or a little something, like crackers, before getting up in the morning.

(6) **Drink plenty of fluids,** especially water and juices. Many doctors recommend pregnant women drink at least **eight glasses of water each day.** More fluids are needed during pregnancy in order to support the increase in the mother's blood volume and maintain the amniotic fluid surrounding the baby. Increased fluid intake also helps prevent constipation. Avoid caffeinated drinks like coffees, teas, or colas. Avoid, too, all alcoholic beverages.

INSTRUCTIONS: Write down *everything* you ate in the last 24 hours.

Breakfast:

Snack:

Lunch:

Snack:

Dinner:

Snack:

Now, using the foods you have listed on this page, fill in ONE DAY of the Diet Chart on the following page. This will help you evaluate how well you are eating for pregnancy, and what foods you may not be eating enough of.

DIET WORKSHEET

(WEEK STARTING_____)

FOOD GROUP	SUNDAY		MONDAY		TUESDAY		WEDNESDAY	
	Daily Servings		Daily Servings		Daily Servings		Daily Servings	
	1 2 3 4 5		1 2 3 4 5		1 2 3 4 5		1 2 3 4 5	
Protein Foods	☐☐☐☐		☐☐☐☐		☐☐☐☐		☐☐☐☐	
Milk & Milk Prod.	☐☐☐☐ +☐*		☐☐☐☐ +☐*		☐☐☐☐ +☐*		☐☐☐☐ +☐*	
Breads & Cereals	☐☐☐☐		☐☐☐☐		☐☐☐☐		☐☐☐☐	
Vitamin C Friuts & Vegs	☐		☐		☐		☐	
Dk. green leafy & yellow Fruits & Vegs	☐☐		☐☐		☐☐		☐☐	
Other Fruits & Vegs	☐☐		☐☐		☐☐		☐☐	

FOOD GROUP	THURSDAY		FRIDAY		SATURDAY	
	Daily Servings		Daily Servings		Daily Servings	
	1 2 3 4 5		1 2 3 4 5		1 2 3 4 5	
Protein Foods	☐☐☐☐		☐☐☐☐		☐☐☐☐	
Milk & Milk Prod.	☐☐☐☐ +☐*		☐☐☐☐ +☐*		☐☐☐☐ +☐*	
Breads & Cereals	☐☐☐☐		☐☐☐☐		☐☐☐☐	
Vitamin C Friuts & Vegs	☐		☐		☐	
Dk. green leafy & yellow Fruits & Vegs	☐☐		☐☐		☐☐	
Other Fruits & Vegs	☐☐		☐☐		☐☐	

Check off for the week: Liver ☐ (1 serving)

* For Pregnant Teenagers or Breastfeeding Moms

Make copies of this page to keep track of your diet.

FOOD GROUPS AND SERVINGS

- **PROTEIN SERVINGS**—Meats, fish, eggs, beans, seeds, and nuts make up the protein food group. For meats, a serving size on the chart would be TWO OUNCES. A quarter pound hamburger (4 ounces) would be two protein servings. A chicken drumstick usually contains about 2 ounces of meat (1 serving), while half a chicken breast contains about 4 ounces of meat (2 servings). Three-quarters of a cup of cooked beans, *1/2 cup of nuts or seeds, or *1/4 cup of nut-butter (4 tablespoons) make one protein serving.

- **MILK AND MILK PRODUCTS**—Milk, cheese, cottage cheese, yoghurt, kefir, and *ice cream make up this food group. One serving of milk or yogurt would be 1 cup (8 ounces). One cheese serving would be about a 1 1/2-inch cube, or about 1 1/2 slices.

- **BREADS AND CEREALS**—Breads, cereals, grains (rice, bulgur, oats, cous-cous), pastas, tortillas, muffins, bagels, buns, and rolls make up this food group. One serving would be one slice of bread, 1/2 English muffin, 1/2 bagel, 1/2 cup of cooked rice, pasta, or hot cereal (like oatmeal or cream of wheat), or 3/4 cup dry cereal (like corn flakes or raisin bran). *Three corn* tortillas or one flour tortilla would make two servings from this food group.

- **VITAMIN C FRUITS AND VEGETABLES**—This food group includes tomatoes, all citrus fruits (oranges, grapefruits, lemons, pineapples), strawberries, and guavas. Eat them fresh and raw whenever possible, as heat or exposure to air will destroy the vitamin C in the fruit (or fruit juice). One serving would be one medium-sized piece of fruit, about 4 ounces of fruit juice, or 3/4 cup of strawberries.

*These foods are high in fat.

- **DARK GREEN LEAFY OR YELLOW FRUITS AND VEGETABLES**—Iceberg lettuce is NOT dark green! Romaine, spinach, chard, kale, bok choy, brussel sprouts, and asparagus are some examples of *dark* greens. Eat at least half of your greens each week raw, in salads.

  Yellow fruits and vegetables include apricots, nectarines, and peaches, as well as yams, sweet potatoes, carrots, yellow and orange squash, and pumpkin. Also included in this group are papayas and mangoes. One serving size would be about 1 cup cooked, or 3/4 cup raw of any of the above.

- **OTHER FRUITS AND VEGETABLES**—Other fruits and vegetables would include any not falling easily into the other groups. This group includes such fruits as apples, bananas, plums, pears, and figs, and such vegetables as potatoes, beets, turnips, corn, green beans, peas, and squash that are *not* yellow or orange. One serving would be one medium-sized piece of fruit, or 1 cup raw or 3/4 cup cooked of any of the above.

Note: These dietary recommendations have been adapted by Christine L. Vega, M.P.H., R.D., from the State of California Department of Health W.I.C. Program (Women, Infants, and Children supplemental feeding program) guidelines.

INDEX

cola drinks, 63, 117
cold flashes. *See* transition, signs of.
colic, 113
colostrum (the first milk), 101
complaints of pregnancy, 57
conception, 25, 27, 28
confusion. *See* transition, signs of.
constipation, 109, 116, 117
contractions
    of labor, definition, 69
    purpose of, in 1st stage labor, 76
    sign of 1st stage of labor, 74
    nature of, in 1st stage labor, 76, 78
    painful. *See* transition, signs of.
    pushing (2nd stage labor), 71
    3rd stage labor, 92
    after childbirth, 108
cramping, 53
crowning, 88

D

diabetes of pregnancy, 68
diaphragm, 42-45
diet, 35, 38, 56-59, 116-121
dilation. *See* cervix, 1st stage labor (dilation).
drugs, 61, 62
    prescription, 63
drugs while breastfeeding, 108

E

edema, 54, 66
effacing. *See* cervix, thinning of.
egg, 22-27
embryo, 26, 28
exercise, 51, 57
    aerobic, 53

F

fainting, 107
Fallopian tubes, 22-26
fats, 58, 116, 120

fertilization. *See* conception.
fetus, 28-33
fever, 110
fundus
    definition, 94
    massage of, 94, 95

H

heart, 42, 43, 45
heartburn. *See* indigestion.
hemorrhoids, 53
heroin, 63
hiccupping. *See* transition, signs of.
hot flashes. *See* transition, signs of.

I

implantation, 26
incontinence, 49
indigestion, 116, 117
intestines, 42-45
involution, 96
irritability. *See* transition, signs of.

J

jaundice, 102
jogging, 53
junk foods, 57, 59

K

Kegel, Dr. Arnold, 48
kegel muscle, 48-51
kicking (of the baby), 30

L

La Leche League, 114
labor, 1st stage
    definition, 69-71
    easier, 57
    false, 73, 74
    length of, 77
    signs of, 72-75

slowing of, 54
labor, 2nd stage, 82, 85-90
labor, 3rd stage, 91, 92
liver, 42-45

M

medication, 62, 63
menstrual blood, 24, 26
menstruation, 21, 24
morning sicknes. *See* nausea.
mother, the first week
   the blues, 103
   diet, 109
   excessive perspiration, 110
   need for rest, 103, 104
   stresses, 103, 104
mucous plug
   definition, 41
   loss of, 72-74

N

nausea, 84, 117
navel, 100
newborn, 36, 98
   appearance of, 98
   bed for, 102
   bowel movements of, 101
   weight loss, 101
nutrition. *See* diet.

O

ova, 22
ovaries, 22-26
ovulation, 22, 23, 27, 28

P

P.C. muscle, 48-51
P.C.P., 63
pelvis, 20, 48
period (menstrual), 22-24, 26, 28, 36,
  105

placenta, 41, 91, 92, 94, 96, 105
poisons, 60
pre-eclampsia, 68
pregnancy
   start of, 28
   comfort in, 57
prenatal care, 64-68
preservatives, 60
processed foods, 58
protein, 35, 119, 120
pubococcygeus muscle. *See* P.C.
  muscle.
pubic bone, 19, 46, 47
pushing contractions, 83
pushing out the baby, 50, 78, 81-90
   effective position for, 86
   how it works, 87
pushing out the afterbirth, 92

R

rectum, 18, 53, 91, 93, 96
relaxation in 1st stage labor, 76, 77
rooming in, 99
running, 53

S

sedatives, 63
sexual intercourse, 27, 51, 96, 105
sexual response, 51
sleeping, positions for, 54, 55
smoking, 63
sperm, 25, 27
spine, 19, 20, 83
stitches, care of, 108
stomach. *See* abdomen.
sweets, 58
swelling, legs & feet, 54, 68
swimming, 53

T

tail bone, 19, 83
tampons, 96, 105

tea, 63, 117
tiredness, 53, 54
tobacco, 63
tranquilizers, 63
transition
 definition, 82, 83
 signs of, 84
trembling. *See* transition, signs of.

U

umbilical cord, 41, 92, 92, 100
urethra, 18
urine samples, 66
uterus
 definition, 18
 and ovulation, 22-24
 and conception, 25-27
 growth of, 39-47, 54, 66
 P.C. muscle suport of, 48, 49
 1st stage labor, 69-71, 74, 77
 in transition, 82, 83

2nd stage labor, 85, 87
3rd stage labor, 91-95
after childbirth, 96, 97, 105-108

V

vaginia, 81, 23-26, 48, 51
vaginal bleeding, 53, 105-107
vaginal exams, 79-81
varicose veins, 53
vomiting. *See* transition, signs of.

W

walking, 53
water bag. *See* amnion.
water bag, breaking of. *See* amnion,
 breaking of.
weight gain, 59, 66
wine, 63
womb, 18, 22, 39, 41
 See also uterus.